I0429447

PRESENT-DAY GEMS OF THE KINGDOM OF GOD:

JESUS MESSIAH LIVES ON

PRESENT-DAY GEMS OF THE KINGDOM OF GOD : JESUS MESSIAH LIVES ON

COMMENCED WRITING FEBRUARY 2011.

FINISHED WRITING NOVEMBER 2015.

BY ERMINIO TAMPONI

ACKNOWLEDGMENTS

WITH GRATEFUL THANKS I DEDICATE THIS BOOK TO
OUR LORD AND SAVIOUR JESUS IMMANUEL GOD WITH
US, WHO HAS CONTINUALLY PROTECTED AND SAVED ME
FROM ALL EVILS AND DEVILS THROUGHOUT MY LIFE; TO
HIM BE ALL GLORY FOR EVER AND EVER, AMEN!

TO MY CHURCH KENSINGTON TEMPLE HERE IN LONDON,
WHICH HAS BEEN AND CONTINUES TO BE A PLACE OF
NOURISHMENT, RESTORATION AND GUIDANCE.

TO MY FAMILY BACK IN ITALY: TO MY MOTHER CHIARA,
AND TO MY BROTHERS AND SISTER MATTEO, MICHELE
AND MARIA GINA, WHO HAVE AND ARE ASSISTING MY
MOTHER IN HER INVALIDITY AND OLD AGE [89], DURING
MY MISSIONARY ABSENCE HERE IN LONDON.

TO MY SECULAR WORK PLACE: SAN MIGUEL RESTAURANT
IN GREENWICH/LONDON AND ITS TEAM, ESPECIALLY ITS
DIRECTORS: GRATEFULLY TO TEV AND ABDU/HARRY
ABDURAHMAN; ALSO TO ITS HEAD CHEF CARLOS
QUEIROS; ALL OF WHOM I HAVE ALWAYS APPRECIATED,

AND THEY HAVE ALWAYS RESPECTED MY MISSIONARY CALLING.

LOVE AND THANKS TO ALL, ERMINIO

===

PRESENT-DAY GEMS OF THE KINGDOM OF GOD:

JESUS MESSIAH

LIVES ON

CONTENTS

ACKNOWLEDGMENTS

CONTENTS

CHAPTERS:

==================================

1   INTRODUCTION

FEBRUARY - 2011

AS I BEGIN TO WRITE THIS BOOK, MY PRAYER IS THAT BY
GOD'S GRACE ITS READERS SHALL BE ENCOURAGED AND
EDIFIED IN THEIR LIVES AND MINISTRIES (EPH. 4:7-13);
THAT THIS BOOK SHALL HELP YOU, IF AND WHEN IN LINE
WITH THE SCRIPTURES, TO UNDERSTAND THE BIBLE
MORE, AND THAT YOU MAY BE ABLE TO RECIEVE AND
IMPART MORE ITS BLESSINGS TO OTHERS. THE BIBLE IS

THE BEST MODELLING MENTOR ALWAYS AVALAIBLE FOR
US.

I COME FROM A VILLAGE IN THE ITALIAN ISLAND OF
SARDINIA.
I WAS BORN IN 1962 IN A FAIRLY CHRISTIAN CATHOLIC
FAMILY AND ENVIRONMENT.
ALREADY AS A YOUNG TEENAGER, BECAUSE OF THE
COMING OF JESUS, I COULD NOTICE GOD'S GRACE
AROUND US; BUT AT THE SAME TIME I COULD SEE THAT
THINGS COULD HAVE BEEN BETTER THAN WHAT THEY
WERE.
WHAT I MEAN IS THAT BOTH THE CHURCH AND SOCIETY
SHOULD HAVE EXPERIENCED AND REFLECTED MORE OF
THE GRACE OF GOD BECAUSE OF BEING IN THE AGE OF
THE CHURCH: THAS IS HAVING THE PRIVILEGE OF
EXPERIENCING THE PRESENCE OF THE HOLY SPIRIT AND
SO IN CERTAIN DEGREES THE KINGDOM OF GOD AMONG
US, THOUGH NOT FULLY YET [MATTH. 3:2; LUKE 11:20].
THUS THERE WAS NOT THE DUE DESIRE FOR THE
PRESENCE OF GOD.

WHAT WERE THEN THE MAIN PROBLEMS?

IN APRIL 1983 I DECIDED TO COME TO LONDON WITH THE
MAIN PURPOSE OF LEARNING FROM LIFE THERE.
AFTER TEN YEARS IN LONDON, AROUND 1993 I BEGAN TO
VISIT AND ATTEND CHURCHES OF OTHER
DENOMINATIONS TOO; AND IN DECEMBER OF THE SOME

YEAR I ENTERED A CHURCH IN EAST LONDON THAT
SOUNDED LIKE A DISCO FROM THE OUTSIDE.

I WAS THE ONLY NATIVE-EUROPEAN-LOOKING PERSON
AMONG ABOUT 200 AFRICAN MEMBERS MOSTLY
DRESSED IN THEIR TRADITIONAL CLOTHES.
THE PASTORS THERE WELCOMED ME, SHOWED ME THE
SCRIPTURE IN ROMANS 10, THEN HE LAYED HIS HANDS
ON ME AND AS I RENEWED MY CONFESSION OF FAITH, I
FELT A SUBSTANTIAL FILLING OF THE HOLY SPIRIT WITHIN
ME.
THIS WAS WITHOUT DOUBT AN EXPERIENCE THAT HAD A
PROFOUND IMPACT AND INFLUENCE IN MY BOTH
CHRISTIAN AND SECULAR LIFE, A GRACE THAT ALSO
FROM ME TOUCHED OTHERS AROUND ME.

A FEW YEARS AGO' HERE IN LONDON, I HAD THE
PLEASURE TO PERSONALLY MEET AND SHAKE HANDS
WITH A FAMOUS PREACHER AT ALL SOULS CHURCH IN
CENTRAL LONDON: JOHN STOTT, WHO PASSED AWAY
JUST A FEW WEEKS AGO' FROM TODAY AS I AM WRITING.
RIGHT NOW I ONLY REMEMBER THAT HE HAD CALLED ME
"BROTHER ". I WANTED TO GREET HIM, AS I HAD READ
SOME MATERIAL FROM HIS BOOKS DURING MY STUDIES.
INDEED I APPRECIATE THIS MAN'S INTERNATIONAL
FOCUS IN THE MINISTRY!

AGAIN WHAT THEN WERE THE MAIN PROBLEMS IN MY
NATIVE ENVIRONMENT, AS WELL AS ALL OVER THE

WORLD TODAY IN THE CHRISTIAN CONTEXT? IT WAS IN THESE YEARS OF 93-95, ATTENDING DIFFERENT DENOMINATIONS, THAT I BEGAN TO QUESTION WITHIN MYSELF, AND REALISE WETHER FOR A GOOD PART THESE PROBLEMS WERE SOMEHOW TO BE ASSOCIATED WITH CERTAIN CHRISTIAN TRADITIONS WHICH WERE PROBABLY NOT GOOD AND EDIFYING FOR THE CHRISTIAN LIFE IF NOT BASED ON THE SCRIPTURE. AND EVEN TODAY THE UNIVERSAL CHURCH MUST BE VERY AWARE OF JESUS' WORDS OF REBUKE "THUS YOU HAVE MADE THE COMMANDMENT OF GOD OF NO EFFECT BY YOUR TRADITION "[MATTH. 15:6]. BUT CERTAINLY NOT BEING THE JUDGE OF ANYTHING, EVEN TODAY I LET THE SCRIPTURES DO THE JUDGEMENT, AND THESE SCRIPTURES LET THOSE WHO HAVE EARS HEAR [REV. 22].

WITHOUT DOUBT IF WE MIX MAN-MADE TRADITIONS WITH HIS WORD, AND NOT IN LINE WITH IT, THESE MAY BECOME STRANGE GOSPELS, AND SO CAUSE A LOT OF FOG BETWEEN GOD'S VISION TO ABRAHAM AND US HIS CHILDREN.

GOING BACK BRIEFLY TO MY EARLY YEARS IN SARDINIA, I RECEIVED MY APOSTOLIC CALLING AS A YOUNG TEENAGER AS I WAS WALKING NEARBY THE CHURCH OF MY VILLAGE PERHAPS IN 2 DIFFERENT OCCASIONS WITH 2 SIMILAR MESSAGES. BASICALLY A VOICE IN THE AIR HAD TOLD ME IN THE ENGLISH LANGUAGE TO PREACH THE GOSPEL ..., WITH THE STRESS ON JESUS' EAGERNESS TO COME BACK ON EARTH. I HAD CLEARLY UNDERSTOOD THE MESSAGE DESPITE MY THEN LITTLE KNOWLEDGE OF

THE ENGLISH LANGUAGE, AND THIS MESSAGE WAS
REVIVED IN MY LATER YEARS HERE IN LONDON IN MY
MIND AND SPIRIT, ESPECIALLY AFTER BEEN FILLED WITH
THE HOLY SPIRIT IN 1993.

THINGS HOWEVER DID NOT GO SO SMOOTHLY AFTER
THAT, AS THAT MESSAGE MUST HAVE BEEN HEARD ALSO
BY DEMONIC SPIRITS. IN THIS PARTICULAR AND
PERSONAL CONTEXT OF MINE: THAS IS BECAUSE OF MY
YOUNG AGE, MY LTTLE KNOWLEDGE OF THE SCRIPTURES,
NOT BEING FILLED WITH THE HOLY SPIRIT JET, AND FOR
THE ABOVE MENTIONED, VERY LIKELY PROBLEMATIC AND
QUESTIONABLE STATE OF THE CHRISTIAN
ENVIRONMENT, INCLUDING MY SINFUL NATURE ALSO, IT
WAS MORE DIFFICULT FOR ME TO DEFEND MYSELF FROM
 DEMONIC ACTIVITY AGAINST ME, IN ORDER TO
FRUSTRATE GOD'S PURPOSE THROUGH MY
LIFE. MOREOVER I THINK THE ELEMENT OF STRONG
PRAYERS, BOTH IN A NATURAL LANGUAGE AS WELL AS IN
TOUNGES, DID NOT SEEM TO BE FERVENT, TO SAY THE
LEAST. HOWEVER ALL KINDS OF PRAYERS ARE CRUCIAL
FOR THE BELIEVER, AND PRAYER PLAYS A VERY
IMPORTANT PART OF OUR LIFE! MOREOVER WE KNOW
THAT PRAYERS HAVE POWER TO CHANGE OUR HEARTS AS
IN ACTS 4:31 < AND WHEN THEY HAD PRAYED, THE PLACE
WHERE THERE WERE ASSEMBLED TOGETHER WAS
SHAKEN; AND THEY WERE ALL FILLED WITH THE HOLY
SPIRIT, AND THEY SPOKE THE WORD OF GOD WITH
BOLDNESS. >

ANYHOW IT IS NOT THE PURPOSE OF THIS BOOK TO MENTION ALL THE DETAILS OF WHAT HAPPEN NEXT.

BUT BASICALLY DUE TO MY SPIRITUAL PROBLEMS ALSO I HAD TO LEAVE SCHOOL AT THE AGE OF 15, WORK FOR SOMETIMES IN MY FAMILY FACTORY, AT THE AGE OF 17 I WAS TAKEN TO A " SPIRITUAL" INSTITUTION IN ROME AND AFTER 12 DAYS THERE, IN A SMALL ROOM THE " PASTOR/PROFESSOR" IN FRONT OF ME TOLD HIS COLLEAGUES THAT I WAS HOPELESS AND THE ONLY POSSIBLE SOLUTION FOR ME WAS ELECTRICAL, [MY COMMENT: RATHER THAN SPIRITUAL!]. I THOUGHT THAT THESE PEOPLE WERE CRAZY! BUT HOWEVER HAVING HEARD MY FATHER, WHO HAD COME TO VISIT ME, TELLING MY MOTHER ON THE PHONE THAT THUS THEY HAD LOST A SON, I JUST ENTRUSTED MY SPIRIT TO GOD REGARDING THE POSSIBLE FUTURE EVENTS. HOWEVER WITH GOD'S BLESSINGS I WAS TAKEN AWAY BEFORE ANY ELECTRICAL PLUG WOULD COME NEAR ME.

WELL I AM SURE YOU WOULD AGREE WITH ME THAT THESE WORDS ABOVE THAT I HAD HEARD SPOKEN TO ME AND ABOUT ME WERE NOT CERTAINLY THE BEST FOR ANYONE AT ANY AGE, AND ESPECIALLY FOR A SEVENTEEN YEARS OLD YOUNG MAN. WE ALL KNOW THAT IN THE SCRIPTURES WORDS ARE VERY IMPORTANT; AND FOR THE LORD HIS WORDS WERE SPIRIT AND LIFE [JOHN 6:63].

MOREOVER PROV. 18:21 SAYS < DEATH AND LIFE ARE IN
THE POWER OF THE TONGUE, AND THOSE WHO LOVE IT
WILL EAT ITS FRUIT >.

I, WE AND THE WORLD NEEDED AND STILL NEEDS HIS
WORDS IN ALL HIS POWER, TO PRODUCE ALL KIND OF
GOOD FRUIT IN OUR LIVES!

BACK IN SARDINIA I DID NOT WORK AGAIN IN MY FAMILY
FACTORY AND AFTER COMING BACK FROM ONE YEAR OF
MILITARY SERVICE IN 1981-1982, I STARTED TO
TRAVEL...FINALLY IN APRIL 1983 HERE I WAS IN LONDON .

NOW MANY PEOPLE IN LONDON KNOW THAT THIS CITY IS
NOT DEMON FREE!

AND SO IN 1987, AFTER SUFFERING OF OFTEN DEEP
SPIRITUAL DEPRESSION FOR ABOUT TEN YEARS, WITH
JUST ENOUGH MONEY I DECIDED TO GO TO INDIA IN
ORDER TO FIND THE WILL OF LIVING, OR DYE THERE .

I SPENT 5 WEEKS THERE AND NEPAL, AND THOUGH I HAD
NOT FOUND THE WILL OF LIVING THAT I WAS LOOKING
FOR, I CERTAINLY CONCLUDED THAT IT WAS BETTER TO
COME BACK TO LONDON RATHER THAN LET MYSELF DYE
THERE OF HUNGER AND THIRST.

TO MAKE THIS TRIP MORE INTERESTING IT WAS ALSO THE
FACT THAT JUST BEFORE COMING BACK, BECAUSE I THINK

I HAD LOST ALMOST 15 KILOS AND MY PANTS WERE LOOSE, I WAS ROBBED OF MY RETURN TICKET AND THE LITTLE MONEY LEFT.

WHILE WAITING FOR ANOTHER TICKET FROM MY FAMILY, I WAS TRAVELLING WITH A CERTIFICATE FROM THE POLICE STATION TO EXEMPT ME FROM PAYING BUS AND TRAIN FARES.

NOW AS I LOOK BACK TO THAT TIME, I REALISE EVEN MORE THAT I WAS TRAVELLING EMPTY, NOT ONLY OF MONEY, BUT ALSO OF LIFE, OF FAITH AND A PERSONAL INTIMATE RELATIONSHIP AND KNOWLEDGE OF GOD AS MY FATHER

ANYHOW HAVING GONE TO A CONSULATE, I WAS FIRST ASKED TO SIT DOWN AND AFTER 2 HOURS, I WAS TOLD THAT THE INDIAN POLICE WAS LOOKING FOR ME IN RELATION OF DEALING WITH DRUGS, THOUGH I DID NOT EVEN SMOKE CIGARETS .

FINALLY THE ITALIAN CONSULATE WAS HELPFUL AND GAVE ME $5 TO HELP ME WHILE WAITING FOR MY TICKET AND TRAVELLING BACK IN LONDON.

BY THE WAY, SOME DAYS BEFORE I HAD BEEN IN GOA TO SEE THE SEASIDE, WHICH I LIKED; THERE I HAD ALSO SEEN AN EMPTY WOODEN CROSS ERECTED ON THE SAND, WHICH, DESPITE ALL WHAT WAS HAPPENING TO ME, AND

MY ANGER AND DELUSION, IT SERVED ME AS A REMINDER.

THE LAST " INDIAN " STORY THAT I WOULD LIKE TO TELL YOU IS THAT IN THE BUS TRAVELLING TO THE AIRPORT, ITS CONDUCTOR WAS NOT SATISFIED WITH SEING THE DOCUMENT FROM THE POLICE EXCLUDING ME FROM PAYING FARES HAVING BEEN ROBBED OF ALL MY MONEY, SO HE ASKED ME TO PAY FOR MY ROCKSACK! SO BECAUSE I REFUSED, HE TRIED TO MAKE ME GET OFF TWO STOPS BEFORE THE AIRPORT.

IN JUNE 1987 I HAD TO START MY LIFE AGAIN HERE IN LONDON WITH ONLY 2/3 DOLLARS, A PASSPORT AND NOTHING ELSE! WELL IT WAS BETTER THAN NOTHING, WAS NOT IT?

BY THE WAY, AFTERWARDS BACK IN LONDON, A PRIEST HAD LENT ME £20 WHICH I WAS ABLE TO GIVE BACK TO HIM AFTER A FEW WEEKS, AND WHEN I DID I ALSO RECEIVED A " SMACK OF AFFECTION " FROM HIM, THOUGH I AM STILL TRYING TO UNDERSTAND WHY, ACTUALLY I THINK I KNOW NOW! ALSO A FRIEND HAD LENT ME SOME MONEY TOO.

MAY THE LORD BLESS THEM ALL AS THERE WERE VERY IMPORTANT FINANCIAL SEEDS SOWN IN MY LIFE.

WITH GOD'S GRACE I CONTINUED TO WORK IN THE CATERING BUSINESS, AND IT WAS PERHAPS IN 1994 THAT

I STARTED TO ATTEND MY STILL PRESENT CHURCH: KENSINGTON TEMPLE IN CENTRAL LONDON, AND IN LINE WITH GOD'S CALLING WITH MY LIFE, BEING PLEASED WITH THE LIFE WITH THIS CHURCH, BETWEEN 1995 AND 1999, I WAS ABLE TO SUCCESSFULLY COMPLETE A CERTIFICATE AND 2 DIPLOMAS IN CHRISTIAN MINISTRIES AND STUDIES, AS WELL AS WELL WORKING.

BY 2005 I HAD ALSO COMPLETED A BA HONS IN THEOLOGY, AND BY NOV. 2007, I HAD COMPLETED A 7 YEARS TERM OF SERVICE AS A PASTOR IN A SATELLITE CHURCH OF OURS: "TOWER CHRISTIAN CENTRE " WITH MAINLY MEMBERS FROM SIERRA LEONE, THAT IS FROM DEC.-2000 TO NOV.-2007.

WE HAD PRE-PLANTED THIS CHURCH FROM BIBLE COLLEGE IN 99, THEN AFTER ONE YEAR I HAD JONED MY COLLEGUE PASTOR AND HIS WIFE, WHO ARE STILL ITS MAIN PASTORS THERE TODAY. WHAT DOES THIS MEAN? IT MEANS THAT SINCE GOD IS A GOD OF ACTION AND CREATION, SO MUST HIS PEOPLE BE PEOPLE OF ACTION AND CREATIVE, THAT IS A PEOPLE OF MISSION! IN FACT TOUGH WE CAN NEVER UNDERSTAND ALL THE RICHES THAT ARE REFLECTED IN THIS RELATIONSHIP WITHIN THE TRINITARIAN NATURE OF GOD; WE MUST NOT MISS THE FACT THAT THE SCRIPTURES SHOW US JESUS AS SON, WHO WAS NOT JUST IN A RELATIONSHIP OF OBEDIENCE AND TRUST, BUT ALSO OF MISSION!

IT WAS IN SEPTEMBER 2001, AFTER 9 MONTHS THERE, THAT TO MY DEEP DISTRESS AND SHOCK ONE EVENING IN

THE MAIN CHURCH, THAT THE HOLY SPIRIT ASKED ME TO LEAVE SAYING TO APOSTLE CHARLES ABRAHAM FROM NIGERIA WHO WAS ON THE STAGE < IF HE LEAVES, I WILL MAKE HIM ... >; THAT IS: "HE PROMISED ME AN IMPORTANT POSITION" IN THE MAIN CHURCH KENSINGTON TEMPLE.

THEN I HAD TO LEAVE THIS CHURCH AND SPEND ABOUT SIX MONTHS PREACHING IN THE STREETS ON SUNDAY MORNINGS, AND IN MARCH OF THE FOLLOWING YEAR I WENT BACK TO THE SATELLITE CHURCH TO ACQUIRE MORE PASTORAL EXPERIENCE.

HAVING SO LEFT THE SATELLITE CHURCH IN NOV. 2007, I MOVED BACK TO THE MAIN CHURCH TO CONCENTRATE MY CHRISTIAN WORK IN A MORE COSMOPOLITAN CONTEXT ACCORDING TO MY CALLING, AND IN FAITH AND OBEDIENCE TO GOD'S DIRECTION AND PREVIOUS MESSAGE. ONE YEAR LATER IN AUGUST I JOINED ITS MINISTRY TEAM OF WHICH I AM PART STILL TODAY, AND THROUGH WHICH ALSO GOD HEALS MANY PEOPLE BEFORE OUR VERY EYES. I GUESS THAT WE, THE MISSIONARY CHURCH, CAN AND SHOULD GO ONLY WHERE OUR LORD JESUS WHO WAS AND STILL IS BY HIS HOLY SPIRIT AND US HIS " BODY " THE MISSIONARY PER EXCELLENCE, WANTS US TO GO; SO THAT WE CAN ALSO AIM AT RECIEVING HIS EXCELLENCE GRACE, AND SO BRINGING GOOD FRUIT TO HIM [JOHN 15].

I THINK JOHN 15:7 IS A GOOD VERSE TO MEMORISE AND MEDIDATE UPON AS THE LORD ENCOURAGE US < "IF YOU ABIDE IN ME, AND MY WORDS ABIDE IN YOU, YOU WILL ASK WHAT YOU DESIRE, AND IT SHALL BE DONE FOR YOU. >

EVEN TODAY AS I WRITE [24-2-2011], THOUGH I AM STILL WORKING IN THE CATERING BUSINESS, AND I HAVE SO FAR NEVER BEEN FORMALLY EMPLOYED BY ANY CHURCH, I DO NOT HAVE ANY DOUBT THAT GOD WILL KEEP AND PERFORM HIS PURPOSES AND PROMISES IN MY LIFE, DESPITE ALL.

WHILE WAITING TO BE FULLY RELEASED IN THE MINISTRY, I FELT IN MY SPIRIT, IT WAS TIME FOR ME TO WRITE THIS BOOK.

IT IS A SIMPLE BOOK, EASY TO READ AND HOPEFULLY ENTERTAINING TOO, AND AS I SAID ABOVE, IT HAS ALSO THE AIM TO TRY TO BRING BLESSINGS TO ITS READERS. YOU MUST HAVE ALREADY NOTICED IT HAS TO DO ONLY WITH REAL AND PERSONAL EXPERIENCES IN MY CHRISTIAN LIFE AND MINISTRY, AND I BELIEVE THESE ARE JUSTIFIED BY THE BIBLE, BUT BEING HUMAN LIKE YOU, I BEG YOU TO LOOK AT THEM THROUGH THE SCRIPTURES, AS THESE ARE THE ONLY MEASURING ROD OF TRUTH.

PLEASE SEE JOHN 4:14; AND THE LORD JESUS IN JOHN 8:31-32 TELLS THAT < ..."IF YOU ABIDE IN MY WORD, YOU

ARE MY DISCEPLES INDEED. AND YOU SHALL KNOW THE
TRUTH, AND THE TRUTH SHALL MAKE YOU FREE." >.

SO LET US BELIEVERS, AGREE IN PRAYER AS WE READ THIS
LAST VERSE TOGETHER BY SAYING "AMEN "!

===

2 HEAVENLY ACTIVITIES PART A

IN THIS CHAPTER I TRY TO DESCRIBE SOME OF THE EXPERIENCES THAT IN THE LAST 17 YEARS I WAS BLESSED WITH THROUGH THE GRACE OF OUR LORD JESUS CHRIST.

ONCE FILLED WITH THE SPIRIT AT THE END OF 1993, THE PEACE OF GOD WAS MORE INTENSE UPON ME WHEREVER I WOULD BE. BEING ALSO MUCH MORE CONSCIOUS OF HIS PRESENCE WITHIN ME AND WITH THE HELP OF HIS GRACE, THE FOLLOWING YEAR I CUT AWAY

FROM WRONG HABITS THAT WERE DISTURBING ME FROM FOCUSING IN A LIFE OF HOLINESS AND PURITY. I STARTED TO ATTEND THE CHURCH 2-3-4 TIMES A WEEK WITH GREAT JOY, AND THERE ENGAGE IN A LOT OF PRAYER, AND TO MY JOY, TO SPEND HOURS SINGING EVERY WEEK.

I STILL REMEMBER ONE INTERESTING AND PROFOUND DETAIL THAT I HAD NOTICED FROM THIS SPIRITUAL TRANSFORMATION. WHAT REALLY HIT MY ATTENTION WAS THE FACT THAT WHILE AND DURING MY OFTEN WALKS THROUGH KENSINGTON GARDENS, A LARGE PARK NOT FAR FROM OUR CHURCH, THIS TIMES IT LOOKED DIFFERENT TO MY EYES THAN BEFORE. THE TREES WERE MORE BEAUTIFUL TO MY EYES, ALL THE SCENARY SEEMED TO BE MORE PLEASANT, ATTRACTIVE AND ENJOYABLE; AS I OBSERVE IT LOOKED ALMOST WONDERFULTO ME AND I WAS HAPPIER TOO.

EVEN TODAY THIS IS SOMETHING THAT I DO NOT FULLY UNDERSTAND IN ITS IMPLICATIONS; THE NATURAL ENVIRONMENT SEEMED TO BE ALL DIFFERENT TO MY SIGTH, THOUGH BEING THE SAME PLACE!

DID THIS REFLECT A RELATIONSHIP BETWEEN ME AND THE NATURAL ENVIRONMENT THERE IN A MORE RIGHTFUL AND SUITABLE FOR OUR CHRISTIAN LIFE NOW, AND SO A STEP CLOSER TO THE FUTURE REALITIES OF THE MILLENNIUM KINGDOM HERE ON PARADISE ON

EARTH OF GENESIS 2, OR IN THE NEW HEAVEN AND
EARTH?

BEFORE MOVING ON, I BRIEFLY WANT TO STRESS THAT IT
WAS ONLY MY REACTION TO THIS NATURAL
ENVIRONMENT THAT STROKE ME RATHER THAN ANY
REACTIONS TO MAN-MADE BUILDINGS/STREETS, ETC...

PERHAPS IT MAY BE OF USEFUL REFLECTION TO OBSERVE
GOD'S DIRECTIONS TO MOSES FOR THE USE OF UNCUT
STONES IN BUILDING AN ALTAR AFTER THE GIVING OF
THE TEN COMMANDMENTS AS IN EX. 20:25 < 'AND IF
YOU MAKE ME AN ALTER OF STONE, YOU SHALL NOT
BUILT IT OF HEWN STONE; FOR IF YOU USE YOUR TOOL
ON IT, YOU SHALL PROFANE IT. >

AFTER THIS PROFOUND CHANGE IN MY LIFE I SOON
BEGAN TO OUTREACH TO OTHER PEOPLE WITH THE
GOSPEL AS MANY OTHERS DO. I WOULD WITNESS TO
THEM WHENEVER AND WHEREVER I COULD, AND AS
ALREADY MENTIONED IN 95 I STARTED BIBLE COLLEGE.
I BELIEVE WITHOUT DOUBT THAT ALSO BECAUSE OF THIS
ZEAL AND WITNESSING OUT OF HIS CALLING AND GRACE,
THAT I HAVE BEEN THROUGH SO MANY EXPERIENCES
THAT I CAN NOW DESCRIBE IN THIS BOOK. I ALSO BELIEVE
WE CAN NEVER STOP WORSHIPING GOD FOR IS REAL AND
PRACTICAL LOVE THROUGH THE INCARNATION OF HIS
SON.

****

IN THESE YEARS I THINK I HAVE SEEN THE THICK, NOT-SEE-THROUGH, WHITE CLOUD OF THE GLORY OF GOD THREE TIMES. TO MY UNDERSTANDING IN THE OLD TESTAMENT THE WHITE CLOUD WOULD COVER THE SPIRIT OF GOD, OR BETTER IT WAS TAKEN TO BE HIS GLORY AND VERY PRESENCE [EX. 33:9; MATTH. 17:5].

MAY THE LORD HAVE MERCY UPON ME FOR ALL MY MISTAKES AND OFFENCES TO OTHERS AND VICEVERSA; AND IT WAS IN ONE OF THIS OCCASIONS, I BELIEVE IN NEED OF HIS CONFORT AND ENCOURAGEMENT, THAT I HAD THIS EXPERIENCE THE FIRST TIME.

WE WERE IN THE NORTH ACTON TABERNACLE OF KENSINGTON TEMPLE ON A SUNDAY EVENING, WITH USUALLY 2-3 THOUSANDS ATTENDERS,WHEN AT A CERTAIN MOMENT GOD LIFTED MY GAZE AND LOOKING UP IN THE AIR UNDER THE HIGH CEILING, I SAW A MANIFESTATION OF HIM. I REMEMBER THAT I SAW THE SIDE OF HIS FACE ONLY, IF I MAY SAY SO, IN PROFILE. THE MESSAGE THAT I THOUGTH THIS CARRIED FOR ME, WAS AS IF GOD WAS SAYING TO ME TO KEEP GOING AND TO STAY FOCUSED ON HIM, NO MATTER WHAT. NOW THE DIMENSIONS OF THIS MANIFESTED APPEARENCE OF THE PROFILE OF HIS FACE WAS PERHAPS WITHIN A SQUARED METER, LIKE A PERFECT DESIGN OF A PROFILE OF A FACE WITH A PERFECTLY CORRESPONDENT SHAPE OF A NOSE TOO.

I MUST ALSO SAY THAT IN THIS KIND OF REFLECTION OF HIM I PERCIEVED SIGNS OF HIS STRENGTH AND ASSURANCE, IT PORTRAYED NO SIGN OF WEAKNESS, CONFUSION, NOR THAT HE HAD LOST CONTROL OF HIS CREATION AND SALVATION PLAN!

I KNOW IT IS DIFFICULT TO AVOID OFFENCES, OR IMPOSSIBLE AT THE MOMENT, AND SO WE ARE CALLED TO BE PATIENT TOO. HOWEVER AS HIS CHURCH WE MUST ALSO DEFEND HIS WORD OF REVELATION FOR US.

ANYHOW IT WAS FOR ME A BEAUTIFUL EXPERIENCE THAT GAVE ME MORE CONFORT AND ASSURANCE IN HIM TO CARRY ON STAYING FOCUSED ON HIM AS HEBR. 12:1-2 < THEREFORE WE ALSO, SINCE WE ARE SURROUNDED BY SO GREAT A CLOUD OF WITNESSES, LET US LAY ASIDE EVERY WEIGHT, AND THE SIN WHICH SO EASILY ENSNARES US, AND LET US RUN WITH ENDURANCE THE RACE THAT IS SET BEFORE US, LOOKING ON TO JESUS, THE AUTHOR AND FINISHER OF OUR FAITH, WHO FOR THE JOY THAT WAS SET BEFORE HIM ENDURED THE CROSS, DESPISING THE SHAME, AND HAS SAT DOWN AT THE RIGHT HAND OF THE THRONE OF GOD. >

****

NOW IN THESE YEARS IN SERVING THE LORD IN THE WAYS DESCRIBED ABOVE AS WELL AS BEING SECOND PASTOR IN

A SATELLITE CHURCH FOR SEVEN YEARS, I ALSO HAVE BEEN REGURARLY VISITING AND MINISTERING TO PATIENTS IN PSCHIATRIC HOSPITALS. IT IS IN FACT THE OPINION OF MANY THAT SOME THESE PATIENTS HAVE ALSO A SPIRITUAL PROBLEM, SOMETIMES MAINLY, SOMETIMES RELATED WITH PROBLEMS WITH OTHER NATURE SUCH AS CHEMICAL IMBALANCE IN THEIR BRAINS, WHICH CERTAINLY REQUIRES SUITABLE MEDICATIONS. NO DOUBT THE PERSON BEING A SPIRITUAL, MENTAL AND PHYSICAL, UNIT IS AFFECTED BY A CONDITION SUCH AS DEPRESSION, OPPRESSION, AND VARIOUS PSHYCO-RELATED ILLNESSES, IN ALL HIS DIMENSIONS; EACH IN VARIOUS DEGREES ACCORDING TO THE PERSONAL PATHOLOGY AND CONTEXT.

IT WAS IN ONE OF THIS SITUATION, MAYBE ABOUT 13 YEARS AGO', THAT WHILE VISITING AN ITALIAN FRIEND OF MINE IN A "WARD OF PATTERSON WING ", AN EXTENSION OF ST. MARY HOSPITAL, JUST BEHIND IT, IN CENTRAL LONDON, THAT I HAD AN OTHER WONDERFUL ENCOUNTER. THOUGH NOT KNOWING A LOT ABOUT HER, I WAS AWARE THE SHE WAS NOT A COMMITTED BELIEVER, MAYBE JUST A NOMINAL ONE IN FACT, SUFFERED FROM DEPRESSION AND SEXUAL IMMORALITY, AND PERHAPS LIKE MANY WITH A LOT OF FAMILY PROBLEMS.

WE WERE IN THE SITTING ROOM OF THE WARD; VARIOUS KINDS OF PATIENTS WERE THERE, COMING IN AND OUT;

THE CARPET WAS NOT WITHOUT FEW CIGARETTES
BURNS, AS I THINK PATIENTS WERE STILL ALLOWED
TO SMOKE WITHIN AT THAT TIME. AND SO AFTER
HAVING A CHAT WITH HER WE SAT TOGETHER ON THE
SOFA AND I BEGAN TO READ FROM THE BOOK OF
PHILIPPIANS 4 WHERE PAUL ENCOURAGES US TO RECIEVE
PEACE FROM GOD THROUGH PRAYER, RATHER THAN
BEING ANXIOUS IN ANYTHING. SUDDENLY AS I WAS
READING, I SAW RIGHT BEFORE US LIKE THE TOP HALF OF
A PERSON MADE BY A THICK WHITE CLOUD THAT
STOPPED ME FROM SEING THE WALL BEHIND HIM; THIS
WALL WAS JUST PROBABLY NOT EVEN 3 YARDS FROM US!

HE WAS MAYBE JUST WITHIN 2 FEET FROM US, HIS ARMS
WERE STREACHED TOWARDS MY FRIEND, LIKE HE WAS
INVITING HER TO HIM, THERE WAS NO APPEARENCE OF
HIS FACE THOUGH, AND NOT A WORD, APART FROM
"PHILIPPIANS "BEING READ TO HER.

HE SUDDENLY DISAPPEARED. TO MY GREAT IMPACT,
I STILL REMEMBER TODAY THAT IN THE ROOM AFTER HE
LEFT, I FELT A GREAT SENSE OF PEACE AND JOY, SO GREAT
THAT BEFORE LEAVING I FELT THAT I COULD NOT
WAIT TO GO BACK THERE; THE ATMOSPHERE HAD
CHANGED, AS BEFORE WALKING IN, IT HAD SEEMED TO
ME RATHER A DEPRESSIVE PLACE TO BE. I BELIEVE WE
NEED TO PRAY MORE IN ORDER TO HELP PEOPLE IN
OUR EVANGELISTIC GOAL TO GET THESE HAVE AN
INTIMATE RELATIONSHIP WITH JESUS SO THAT THAT TO
SERVE HIM AFTER, VS. TOO MANY THEOLOGICAL DETAILS
AND PRINCIPLES.

IT COMES TO MY MIND NOW JACOB'S REACTIONS AFTER SEEING THE LORD IN A DREAM IN GEN 28:17. YOU MAY LIKE TO KNOW THAT I ASKED THIS PERSON ABOUT THE "VISITATION OF THE LORD ", AND TO MY SURPRISE THEN, SHE TOLD ME THAT SHE NEVER SAW OR NOTICED ANYTHING.

BUT LET US SEE TOGETHER MATTH. 15:5 IN THE TRANSFIGURATION ACCOUNT < WHILE HE WAS STILL SPEAKING, BEHOLD, A WHITE CLOUD OVERSHADOWED THEM; AND SUDDENLY A VOICE CAME OUT OF THE CLOUD, SAYING, "THIS IS MY BELOVED SON, IN WHOM IN WHOM I AM WELL PLEASED. HEAR HIM!" >.

LET US SAY AMEN TO THAT TOO.

****

WELL I THINK THE LAST TIME I SAW THIS " WHITE CLOUD " MANIFESTATION, IT MUST HAVE BEEN ABOUT TEN/TWELVE YEARS AGO'. I WAS IN ITALY ON HOLIDAYS, IN MY PARENTS' HOUSE, AND PEHAPS I WAS STILL IN BIBLE COLLEGE IN LONDON. I REMEMBER WE WERE HAVING DINNER AT HOME IN OUR SITTING ROOM, AND I CAN NOT TELL NOW WHETHER I WAS THINKING TO PRAY FOR A SICK PERSON IN PARTICULAR IN MY VILLAGE, OR

JUST IN A GENERAL CONTEXT; HOWEVER SOMEHOW DOUBTS WERE RISING IN MY MIND REGARDING MY FAITH AND POWER IN THE LORD TO HEAL THE SICK.

SUDDENLY AS I WAS THINKING SO, I FELT LIKE A LITTLE WHITE CLOUD [OR BETTER A BIT OF THE HOLY SPIRIT] HAD COME OUT OF ME AND REMAINED BETWEEN ME AND MY PLATE RIGHT BEFORE ME. QUITE EXTRAORDINARLY AND FUNNY I COULD NOT SEE MY PLATE IN FRONT OF MY FACE! IN FACT I COULD JUST ABOUT NOTICE A SMALL PART OF ITS ROUND EDGE. IN MY REPENTANCE AND SORROW IN DOUBTING, I WAS GREATFUL TO GOD AND KEPT THE MATTER IN MY MIND AND CLEARED IT OF ANY DOUBTS TOO. IN THESE CONTEXTS WE CAN AND SHOULD FIND MUCH COURAGE IN JESUS' WORDS IN MK. 5:36 < ...'DO NOT BE AFRAID; ONLY BELIEVE'. >

****

AS I HAVE ALREDY MENTIONED, I HAVE BEEN PART OF [KENSINGTON TEMPLE] MINISTRY TEAM FOR OVER 2 YEARS; DURING THIS TIME, AND SOMETIMES IN THE PAST, THE LORD HAS USED ME VARIOUS TIMES IN HEALINGS, SUCH AS OF EYES, HEARING AND PAINS. IN PARTICULAR I REMEMBER AN OLD LADY HEALED FROM AN EYE CONDITION, MAYBE A CATARACT; HAVING TOUCHED HER EYES AND PRAYED, AS USUAL I ASKED HER

HOW SHE WAS AND COULD SEE AFTER PRAYER, AND TO MY HAPPINESS AND JOY AND A LITTLE SURPRISE TOO, HER FACE HAD CHANGED AND LOOKED BRIGHTER AND TOLD ME THAT SHE COULD SEE MUCH BETTER. I REMEMBER SHE WAS RATHER EXCITED THAT EVEN HER DENTURE MOVED A LITTLE TOO FORWARD AS SHE OPENED HER MOUTH TO CONFESS HER HEALING TO ME.

AS WELL AS THIS HEALING I ONLY WISH TO DESCRIBE AN OTHER ONE WHICH GOD PERFORMED THROUGH ME, OR RATHER MORE LIKE A MIRACLE.

THIS MUST HAVE HAPPENED ABOUT 10/13 YEARS AGO', I CANNOT REMEMBER WHETHER I WAS STILL IN BIBLE COLLEGE OR NOT, AND WHETHER I HAD STARTED MY PASTORAL WORK IN THE SATELLITE CHUCH; HOWEVER I WAS INVOLVED IN THE 2:30 SERVICE PRAYING FOR PEOPLE AND HELPING TO BAPTISE THEM. IT HAPPENED THAT AMONG THE PEOPLE WHO WERE BAPTISED, THERE WAS A MAN FROM NORTH OF ENGLAND. I WAS TOLD THAT HE HAD JUST GONE THROUGH A SERIES OF COUNSELLING SESSIONS WITH THE CHURCH, AND HAD DECIDED TO BECOME A COMMITTED BELIEVER IN THE LORD JESUS; HIS PAST HISTORY HAD SOMEHOW BEEN ASSOCIATED I THINK WITH DRUGS AND CHILD ABUSE ALSO THOUGH I DO NOT REMEMBER IN WHAT DETAILS.

NOW WE WERE IN THE BASEMENT KITCHEN CHANGING OUR WET CLOTHES FROM THE WATER BAPTISM WITH IMMERSION, JUST PERFORMED UPSTAIRS IN THE TANK UNDER THE STAGE OF THE CHURCH; AS USUALLY AFTER

GETTING CHANGED WE WOULD PRAY FOR EACH BAPTIST CANDIDATE BEFORE LETTING THEM GO.

NOW AS I LOOKED AT THIS PERSON, I NOTICED THAT HE WAS A LITTLE SCARING TO LOOK AT, LIKE HE HAD GONE THROUGH VARIOUS DRAMAS THAT PSYCHOLOGICALLY HAD SCARRED HIM IN HIS LIFE; ALSO HIS EYES SEEMED TO HAVE BEEN NOT IN LINE WITH EACH OTHER, HIS FACE LOOKED SERIOUSLY UGLY AND A LITTLE DEFORMED.

I THOUGTH THAT IN THAT STATE HE WOULD HAVE HAD SOME PROBLEMS IN RELATIONSHIPS, AND SO BEFORE SENDING HIM BACK OUTSIDE, SINCE HE JUST HAD RECIEVED AN INNER AND SPIRITUAL HEALING, I DECIDED THAT IT WAS A GOOD IDEA TO ASK THE LORD TO GIVE HIM AN OUTSIDE TRASFORMATION OF HIS FACE TOO.

TAKING ADVANTAGE OF THE FACT THAT WE HAD SURROUNDED HIM TO PRAY FOR HIM AND BLESS HIM BEFORE HE WENT, JUST FOR A FEW SECONDS I PUT MY HANDS OVER HIS FACE IN FULL CONVICTION IN MY MIND AND SPIRIT, AFTER HAVING TOLD HIM TO STOP MESSING AROUND AND BE FAITHFUL TO THE LORD, AND TO MY MARVEL AND JOY, AFTER TAKING MY HANDS OFF, HIS FACE LOOKED ALMOST LIKE THAT OF AN OTHER PERSON.

THE LORD HAD JUST GIVEN HIM LIKE A "PLASTIC SURGERY ", FREE, INSTANTANOUS AND PERFECT: HE LOOKED HANDSOME AND ATTRACTIVE NOW; EVERY PART OF HIS FACE WAS NOW PERFECTLY PROPORTIONED AND PLACED

IN RESPECT OF THE REST; I FELT THAT HE NEEDED I NEW PASSPORT NOW, BUT THAT WOULD HAVE BEEN CERTAINLY HIS PROBLEM.

TO GOD'S GLORY HE WOULD HAVE NOW FELT MORE ACCEPTED AND WANTED IN HIS RELATIONSHIPS WITH PEOPLE, ESPECIALLY NOW IN HIS NEW ROLE OF SALT AND LIGHT IN SOCIETY.

I HOPE THAT WHAT YOU HAVE JUST READ WILL ENCOURAGE YOU TO BE MORE CONFIDENT, AND TO ASK AND DO THE THINGS WHICH YOUR HEARTS DESIRES IN THE LORD JESUS; THIS IS ALSO HIS WISH AS WE CAN SEE CLEARLY IN JOHN 14:13-14 < "AND WHATEVER YOU ASK IN MY NAME, THAT I WILL DO, THAT THE FATHER MAY BE GLORIFIED IN THE SON."IF YOU ASK ANYTHING IN MY NAME, I WILL DO IT. >

AMEN!

****

WHAT FOLLOWS NOW IS RATHER A PECULAR STORY, BUT I THINK ALSO INERESTING.

THIS MUST HAVE HAPPENED EITHER AT THE END OF MY BIBLE COLLEGE OR SOON AFTER THAT, PERHAPS IN 99-2000.

MOST LIKELY I MUST HAVE BEEN IN BIBLE COLLEGE DURING THE DAY, AND IN THE EVENING AT WORK IN A WEST END RESTAURANT, JUST BY PICCADILLY.

IN THOSE DAYS I CLEARLY REMEMBER I OFTEN USED TO PRAY TO RECIEVE UNDERSTANDING REGARDING THE EVENT OF PENTECOST; TO BE MORE PRECISE I WANTED TO HAVE MORE INSIGHT REGARDING THE FACT THAT THE PEOPLE OF VARIOUS NATIONALITIES WHO WERE AROUND THE DISCEPLES, COULD HEAR THESE WHO WERE JEWS AND BY THE HOLY SPIRIT SPEAKING IN OTHER TOUNGES, IN THEIR NATIVE LANGUAGES [ACTS 2:1-11].

PLEASE OBSERVE CAREFULLY TWO IMPORTANTS POINTS HERE: 1- IN V.4 WE SEE THAT THEY SPOKE IN OTHER TONGUES! 2- IN V.8 WE CAN SEE THAT EACH LISTENER HEARS THEM EACH IN HIS OWN LANGUAGE!

SO WHAT HAPPENED THEN?

AS SOME OF YOU WILL KNOW, AT TIME TOUNGES CAN ONLY BE UNDERSTOOD WHERE THERE IS GIVEN ITS INTERPRETATION BY OTHERS PRESENT MOVING WITH THE GIFT OF INTERPRETRATION. IN OTHER CASES HOWEVER, AS IN THIS, TONGUES CAN BE RECEIVED AS ALREADY UNDERSTANDABLE SPOKEN FOREIGN LANGUAGES BY THE POWER OF THE HOLY SPIRIT; IN ADDITION, FOR SOME BELIEVE THAT THERE IS THE PERSONAL PRAYER IN TOUNGES JUST TO EDIFY OURSELVES IN PRAYER TO GOD THROUGH THE HOLY SPIRIT [1 COR. 12-14].

SOME HELP CAME TO MY SPIRIT IN THIS
FOLLOWING WAY.

NOW IT HAPPENED THAT AT AROUND ONE IN THE
MORNING OR JUST EARLIER, COMING BACK HOME FROM
WORK, AS USUALLY I WAS APPROACHING THE DOOR OF
MY BEDSIT; TO MY SURPRISE AS I WAS PUTTING THE KEYS
IN THE LOCK AND TURNING THEM INTENDING TO OPEN
THE DOOR, SUDDENLY I CLEARLY HEARD A VOICE
COMING FROM WITHIN MY ROOM, NOT FROM MY HEAD,
NOR A SENSATION: < HE IS COMING, HE IS COMING >; IT
SAYED.

IN MY PERPLEXITY AND UNDERSTANDING I THOUGHT
THAT HE COULD NOT HAVE BEEN AN ANGEL AS ANGELS
ARE NOT SCARED OF HUMANS. WITH CURIOUSITY I WENT
IN THE LARGE ROOM AND IN THE WITHIN CONTAINED
SMALL KITCHEN AND OBVIOUSLY NOBODY WAS THERE.

THIS REMAINED A MYSTERY UNTILL ONE OR TWO DAYS
AFTER. STILL LATE AT NIGHT, AS I WAS OPENING THE
DOOR AND ABOUT TO ENTER IN, THOUGH I HAD HEARD
NO VOICE THIS TIME, I SUDDENLY FELT THAT SOMEBODY
WAS IN THE ROOM AND AGAIN HE WAS SCARED.

AS I TURNED MY FACE INTO THE SMALL KITCHEN
SEPARATION IN THE ROOM,

THAT THERE IT WAS: A LITTLE MOUSE WAS RUNNING TO
HIDE BEHIND THE FRIDGE!

MOST LONDONERS KNOW THAT WE ARE NOT ALONE IN THE CITY, BUT OFTEN MICE LIVE AND GO THROUGH ITS HOUSES AND BUILDINGS.

TO ME THE VOICE THAT I HAD HEARD, WAS AS THE HOLY SPIRIT HAD TRANSLATED IN ENGLISH AND [PERHAPS] LIFTED IN THE AIR THE THOUGTH OF THE SPIRIT OF THE SCARED MOUSE, EXPANDING IT; SO REVEALING IT AND ITS PRESENCE TO ME [I DOUBTED THAT HE HAD SPOKEN AS BALAAM' S DONKEY DID [NUM 22:28]; DO REMEMBER THAT I WAS BEHIND THE DOOR WHEN I HAD HEARD IT CLEARLY!

INDEED THE SPIRIT REVEALS THE PERSON [JOHN 14-16].

IT IS OBVIOUS THAT ALSO ANIMALS THINK AND THAT ARE SOMEHOW INTELLIGENT TOO IN THEIR OWN WAYS. ANYHOW I THANKED GOD AS THIS EXPERIENCE GAVE ME MORE INSIGTH BOTH IN THE ISSUE OF TOUNGES COMMUNICATION AS MENTIONED ABOVE AS WELL AS IN GENERAL IN THE WOUNDERFUL NATURAL AND SUPERNATURAL OUTWORKING OF OUR GOD, WHO IS ALSO IS THE GOD OF ALL SPIRITS [ECCL 3;12; ZECH 12:1]. I BELIEVE THIS IS ALSO A VERY HUMBLING STORY THAT REMINDS US, IN THE MIDST OF ALL OUR SERVICE FOR THE SAVIOUR, TO HOLD AN ATTIDUDE AGAINST PRIDE AND ARROGANCE AS GOD IS THE MAIN EVANGELIST/MISSIONARY!

BY THE WAY, JUST TO LET YOU KNOW HOW THIS ENDED, A FEW DAYS AFTER IN THE MIDDLE OF THE NIGHT, THE LITTLE MOUSE WAS WALKING IN THE ROOM NEXT TO MY BED: WELL IT WAS EITHER IT OR ME! I HAD TO GET UP , HAVING PUT ON MY RUNNING SHOES I CHASED IT FOR AN HALF HOUR; FINALLY WITH THE HELP OF AN UMBRELLA AND A CLOTH, I CAUGHT IT, RAPPED IT AND PUT IT OUTSIDE OF THE HOUSE [SORRY, BUT TRUE].

ANYWAY RATHER THAN COMING TO ANY THEOLOGICAL CONCLUSIONS TO WHAT WE JUST SAYED, I WOULD LIKE TO END THIS LITTLE STORY WITH A VERSE FROM THE APOSTLE PAUL IN ROM. 11:33 < OH, THE DEPTH OF THE RICHES BOTH OF THE WISDOM AND KNOWLEDGE OF GOD! HOW UNSEARCHABLE ARE HIS JUDGMENTS AND HIS WAYS PAST FINDING OUT! >

TOUGH HE REVEALS TO US MANY OF HIS WAYS; THIS IS CERTAINLY A GOOD VERSE TO REFLECT UPON, ESPECIALLY IF WE FEEL WE NEED TO BE MORE HUMBLE!

****

THE NEXT IS A BRIEF STORY BUT I HOPE IT WILL STILL EXCITE AND CHALLENGE YOU.

IT MUST HAVE HAPPENED ABOUT AROUND FIFTEEN YEARS AGO'.

WITH AN EVANGELISTIC TEAM FROM KT [OUR CHURCH],
WE WERE SPENDING SOME TIME IN CENTRAL LONDON,
LEICESTER SQ. SINGING, PREACHING AND WITNESSING TO
THE PEOPLE AROUND US, GIVING LEAFLETS ETC... AS
MANY KNOW THIS LONDON SPOT IS USUALLY
FREQUENTED BY ALL KIND OF PEOPLE, AND IN
PARTICULAR TURISTS FROM ALL OVER THE WORLD; SOME
GO EVEN THERE TO ENTERTAIN THE PUBLIC [AND MAKE
SOME MONEY TOO] WITH OPEN AIR SHOWS, DRAWING
CARICATURES ETC.., REALLY THE IDEAL PLACE TO
EVANGELISE! WELL I AM CERTAINLY PROUD OF MANY OF
OUR CHURCH MEMBERS WHO GETS INVOLVED IN THESE
ACTIVITIES.

ANYHOW I REMEMBER THAT AMONG THESE THERE WERE
A GROUP OF YOUNG MUSLIMS TOO, LISTENING AND
IN DIALOGUE WITH US. I REMEMBER THAT PARTICULAR
EVENING WAS FREEZING COLD, TIME HAD MOVED FAST;
BY THEN IT WAS ALREADY OVER TWO IN THE MORNING,
ONLY FEW OF US WERE LEFT AND THE SQUARE HAD
BECOME COMPLETELY DESERTED ESPECIALLY BECAUSE
OF THE COLD. I RECALL THAT I WAS TAKEN UP IN
WITNESSING TO A YOUNG MUSLIM FOR THE LAST HOUR
OR SO. ANYHOW BECAUSE OF THE TIME, AFTER GIVING
OUR LEAFLETS TO THOSE INTERESTED AND RESPECTFULLY
AGREEING AND DISAGREEING IN VARIOUS ISSUES,
SAYING BYE TO ALL, EACH OF US LEFT THE PLACE.

I CAN NOT TELL EXCATLY WHICH DAY THIS WAS,
HOWEVER THE FOLLOWING SUNDAY, I WAS USUALLY IN
KENSINGTON TEMPLE FOR THE EVENING SERVICE.

ONE OF THE ASPECT I LIKE MOST IN THE CHURCH IS THE WORSHIP, AS EVERY SERVICE START WITH A AT LEAST THIRTY MINUTES OF IT.

AND SO THERE I WAS STANDING UPSTAIRS PRAISING THE LORD. AS A WAS JOYOUS IN THE LORD THINKING ALSO OF THAT EVANGELIST EVENING, I STARTED TO JUMP, SOMETHING I DID/DO NOT USUALLY DO, IN MY EXCITEMENT AND SUDDENLY IN PANIC I SCREAMED BECAUSE I FELT THAT I WAS NOT COMING BACK DOWN ON MY FEET. IN FACT I FELT AS SOMEBODY, WHO COULD HAVE BEEN THE HOLY SPIRIT OR MAYBE AN ANGEL, PEHAPS FOR A SECOND OR ALMOST, WAS HOLDING ME IN THE AIR. IT WAS ABSOLUTLELY MARVELLOUS! WHEN WE OBEY THE GREAT COMMISSION ALL HEAVEN REJOICES WITH US, AS WE ARE DOING SOMTHING IMPORTANT.

BUT PLEASE SEE THESE FOLLOWING VERSES: ACTS 2:40-47; LUKE 4:11. NOW LET US END THIS STORY BY LOOKING AT LUKE 15:7: < "I SAY TO YOU THAT LIKEWISE THERE WILL BE MORE JOY IN HEAVEN OVER ONE SINNER WHO REPENTS THAN OVER NINETY-NINE JUST PERSONS WHO NEED NO REPENTANCE. >

RATHER AN INTERESTING COMMENT BY THE LORD, IS NOT IT?

WELL IT WAS CERTAINLY A SPECIAL WORSHIP TIME, AND THEN I REMAINED IN THE REST OF THE SERVICE AS NORMAL.

****

THE FOLLOWING IS AN EXPERIENCE I HAD PROBABLY 7 OR
9 YEARS AGO'.

I MUST SAY I AM A LITTLE RELUCTANT TO DESCRIBE IT;
NEVERTHELESS IT HAS ITS OWN BEAUTY AND VALUE. IT
HAD HAPPENED THAT IM MY PASTORAL WORK, FOR
VARIOUS REASONS SUCH AS ALSO LEARNING IN
PROGRESS AND OUR HUMAN WEAKNESS, THAT I FELT
QUITE OFFENDED BY A PARTICULAR BEHAVIOUR
TOWARDS ME BY AN OTHER PASTOR. OBVIOUSLY WE ARE
CALLED TO BE INTERCESSORS AND NOT ACCUSERS AS THE
DEVIL IS AND WOULD LIKE US TO BE TOO!

THUS I SHALL TRY TO BE AS COINCISE AS POSSIBLE AS
WELL AS AVOIDING SOME PARTICULAR DETAILS.
ANYHOW I HAVE TO SAY THAT I WAS FEELING RATHER
SHOCKED AND OFFENDED BY IT. PLEASE NOTE THAT AN
OFFENCE IS LIKE A STUMBLIMG BLOCK OR A SNARE,
MEANING ALSO THAT THE CONSEQUENCES OF THE
FOLLOWING FALL COULD BE SERIOUS BRUISES AND
INJURIES TOO, AND THESE COULD ALSO BE MIXED WITH
FEELINGS OF BITTERNESS, ANGER AND RESENTMENT;
CERTAINLY NOT AN NICE COCKTAIL FOR ANY PERSON TO
DRINK AND CARRY ON ABOUT HIS WHATSOVER
PROFESSION, WAS IT NOT FOR THE OPPORTUNITY TO LET
ALL THIS POISON BE ABSORBED BY THE BLOOD OF JESUS.

I THOUGHT IN MY MIND THAT DURING THE WEEK HAD DEALED WITH IT IN PRAYER AND FORGIVENESS, AND I AM SURE THAT AT LEAST PARTIALLY IT WAS SO. ANYHOW THE NEXT SUNDAY MORNING AS A WAS GETTING READY TO GO TO CHURCH, I NOTICED THAT THE PRESENCE OF THE SPIRIT OF THE LORD WAS QUITE INTENSE IN MY ROOM; I FELT AS DRAWN TO THE MIDDLE OF THE ROOM, WHICH I DID, AND UNDER HIS ANOINTING I WAS ALMOST LIKE CAUSED TO STAND THERE WAITING ON HIM. I WAS STANDING IN THIS WAY FOR MAYBE 3-5 MINUTES.

DURING THIS TIME I FELT SO IMPACTED BY HIS SPIRIT, QUENCED UNDER HIS ANOINTING AS HE WAS POURING ON ME HIS LOVE, GRACE AND MERCY THROUGH MY SOUL AND SPIRIT UNTILL I FELT THAT ANY SMALL FEELING OF BITTERNESS AND RESENTMENT TOWARDS THIS PARTICULAR PASTOR OF OUR CHURCHES, HAD BEEN COMPLETELY DROWNED AND CONSUMED WITHIN ME BY THE POWER OF HIS OVERWHELMING LOVE AND GRACE TOWARDS US.

IT FOLLOWED THAT IN THE NEXT WEEK THIS PARTICULAR PASTOR WAS MORE SHOCKED BY GOD'S LOVING GRACE THROUGH ME TOWARDS HIM, THAN I HAD BEEN SHOCKED BEFORE BECAUSE OF THE OFFENSE! IT IS ONLY THROUGH HIS GRACE THAT WE CAN KEEP SOME INTEGRITY, AND THIS IS ESSENTIAL, IF WE CHRISTIANS WANT TO ATTRACT OTHERS, SO THAT WE CAN MAKE WAY FOR GOD'S GRACE TO CHANGE THEIR DESTINY.

TO GOD BE THE GLORY THEN, AND AS THE LOVING FATHER OF ALL HIS CHILDREN, IT IS CERTAINLY AT THE CENTRE OF HIS WILL, HIS HEART FELT DESIRE AND CALL FOR UNITY AMONG BELIEVERS AND CHURCHES IN OUR SPIRITS AND MOST OF ALL IN THE HOLY SPIRIT.

 THUS LET US MAKE THE PROPHETIC WORDS OF BOTH THE LORD IN JOHN 17:21, AND OF PAUL IN 2 COR. 3:6, OURS PRAYERS TOO! < "THAT THEY ALL MAY BE ONE, AS YOU, FATHER, ARE IN ME, AND I IN YOU; THAT THEY ALL MAY BE ONE IN US, THAT THE WORLD MAY BELIEVE THAT YOU SENT ME. > AND OF PAUL: < WHO HAS ALSO MADE US SUFFICIENT AS MINISTERS OF THE NEW COVENANT, NOT OF THE LETTER BUT OF THE SPIRIT; FOR THE LETTER KILLS, BUT THE SPIRIT GIVES LIFE. >

I SAY AMEN TO THESE, FOR THE GLORY OF GOD!

======================================
===

3   HEAVENLY ACTIVITIES PART B

AS I CONTINUE WITH MY NARRATIVE OF SOME MAJOR

FACTS IN MY CHRISTIAN LIFE, THE NEXT STORY I WOULD LIKE TO TELL YOU IT HAS A CURIOUS BUSINESS TONE TOO. I HAVE ALREADY MENTIONED IN MY INTRODUCTION THAT FOR MANY YEARS AND STILL NOW, I HAVE BEEN SUPPORTING MY MINISTRY WORKING IN THE CATERING BISINESS. IT HAPPENED HOWEVER THAT ABOUT THREE YEARS AGO' I LEARNED THAT SOME FRIENDS, WHO WERE ALSO WORKING IN CATERING HAD SOME BUSINESS INTERESTS TOO. THESE WERE ACTUALLY TRYING TO ACT AS INTRODUCERS, MEDIATORS OR AGENTS; FUNNY ENOUGH, I WAS KEEN TO BE INVOLVED IN IT.

IN CONNECTION WITH THEM AND OTHER PEOPLE THAT I MET, THINKING ALSO HOW THE LORD JESUS WAS OFTEN IN BOATS AND AMONG FISHERMEN, I BEGAN TO PROMOTE VARIOUS SORTS OF PRODUCTS: GOLD, DIAMONDS, PETROLEUM PRODUCTS, CURRENCIES, EVEN VILLAS, LARGE EXTENSIONS OF LANDS FOR CONSTRUCTIONS, AND SHIPS. AS YOU CAN IMMAGINE I MET VARIOUS KIND OF PEOPLE INVOLVED IN THIS, INCLUDING BEING IN A FEW MEETINGS WITH A VERY WEALTHY SHIPS OWNER. ANYHOW MY STORY HAS TO DO WITH A DEAL IN PETROLEUM. IT HAPPENED THAT ABOUT 2 AND HALF YEARS AGO' DURING A VISIT OF A CHURCH IN CENTRAL LONDON THAT I HAD MET A GENTLEMAM WHO WAS ALSO A MEMBER OF ITS COUNCIL FOR SOME YEARS TOO. TO MY GREAT HAPPINESS THIS WAS A DIRECT AGENT [MANDATE] OF A RUSSIAN REFINERY!

WELL HAVING EXCHANGED DETAILS AND RECIEVED ITS SOFT OFFER WITH ITS PRICES AND PROCEDURES, STRAIGHT AWAY I BEGAN TO PROMOTE THE PRODUCTS: CRUDE, JET

FUEL [JP 54] DIESEL, ECT...

TO INCREASE THE POSSIBILITIES TO MAKE BETTER BUSINESS
CONNECTIONS I ALSO JOINED VARIOUS CASINOS IN THE
WESTEND HERE IN LONDON. IT WAS IN ONE OF THIS,
PRECISLY IN MAY FAIR, THAT I HAD MET A BUSINESS MAN
FROM INDIA. HE WAS OLDER THAN ME, AND SO IT SEEMED
MUCH MORE EXPERIENCED TOO. IT WAS ON A FRIDAY
NIGHT, I HAD JUST LEFT THE CHURCH AND I THOUGHT
GOD'S BLESSINGS WERE ON ME. VERY SOON I TALKED
TO HIM BY THE BAR AND WE WENT TO SIT DOWN
TOGETHER AND BEGAN TO TALK ABOUT THE GOLD OF THE
KING OF THAILAND.

AT THAT TIME I WAS IN FACT IN CONTACT WITH AN AGENT
IN THAILAND WHO WAS PROMOTING THIS GOLD.
INCREDIBLY THIS MAN IN THE CASINO TOLD ME THAT HE
HAD BEEN INVOLVED IN THIS MATTER ABOUT TWENTY
YEARS BEFORE, AND FOR SOME REASONS ADVISED ME
TO NOT TO PURSUE THE MATTER ANY LONGER, WHICH I
DID ALSO DUE TO THE WORSENING OF THE
COMMUNICATIONS BETWEEN ME AND THE PARTIES
INVOLVED.

I REMEMBER HAVING TALKED TO HIM ABOUT THE
PETROLEUM OPPORTINITIES TOO AND I WAS ENCOURAGED
BY HIM. WITH THIS MAN FOR SOME TIME WE EVEN TRIED
TO SELL A 95 MILLIONS EURO YAUGHT, AND SEEMINGLY
FOUND A POTENTIAL BUYER TOO. WELL IT WAS AFTER I
THINK ALMOST 2 YEARS THAT THROUGH HIM I RECIEVED
THE FIRST ORDERS FOR PETROLEUM PRODUCTS, JET FUEL

TO BE MORE SPECIFIC.

I COULD ALMOST NOT BELIEVE MY EYES WHEN I SAW THESE
TWO ICPOS [IRREVOCABLE CORPORATE PURCHASE
ORDERS], WITH ITS ACCOMPANING DOX FOR
COMMISSIONS AND PRIVACY. WITHOUT GOING INTO
DETAILS EACH ORDER WAS BIG ENOUGH TO MAKE ALL THE
AGENTS INVOLVED IN THE DEAL MILLIONAIRS IN A YEAR!
FOR A WHILE AND A FEW TIMES I HAD TO STOP WORKING
AT THE COMPUTER AS I WAS IN A STATE OF SHOCK!

WHAT HAPPENED THEN IS THAT FOR PRUDENCE I SEND AN
EMAIL WITH ONE ORDER ONLY TO MY ASSOCIATE FROM
THE CHURCH, THE REFINERY'S AGENT, CONFIRMING ALSO
WITH HIM THE AGREED PERCENTAGE OF MY
COMMISSIONS.

DURING THESE TWO YEARS I HAD MET WITH HIM AT
VARIOUS TIMES TO DISCUSS DETAILS AND MY
COMMISSIONS; I HAD IN MY HAND MANY DOCUMENTS ON
BOTH HIM AND THE REFINER. ON THE SELLING SIDE IT WAS
JUST HIM AND ME; I ALWAYS KNEW HIM AS ONE COMPANY
AND NEXT TO THE SUPPLIER. IT FOLLOWED THAT I
RECIEVED HIS CALLING LATE IN THE MORNING; OBVIOUSLY
HE WAS VERY HAPPY TO RECIEVE THE ORDER, BUT DENIED
THAT HE HAD AGREED ON THAT PARTICULAR
COMMISSION!!!

I MUST SAY IT WAS NOT A VERY CORDIAL PHONECALL! IT
HAD TAKEN ME 2 YEARS BEFORE RECIEVING THESE ORDERS;
TO MY FURTHER SHOCK IT CONTINUED TO TELL ME THAT

HE WAS NOT ACTING AS ONE COMPANY BUT IN FACT AS THREE COMPANIES!!! MY COMMISSIONS HAD JUST GONE DOWN MUCH FURTHER, AND EVEN WORSE MY TRUST ON HIM TOO! TOO MUCH WAS AT STAKE, SO I TRYED TO RECONCILE MY RAPPORT WITH HIM. PERHAPS SOME OF YOU MAY IDENTIFY WITH MY FEELINGS WHEN I SWITCHED OFF THE PHONE. I HONESTLY THINK THAT I WAS NOT JUST ANGRY BUT ALSO MUST HAVE FELT SOME HATRED TOO AGAINST HIM [SORRY BUT PROBABLY VERY TRUE].

WHAT HAPPENED NEXT WAS QUITE WONDERFUL. AS I TURNED AROUND IN MY DESPARATION, THE WOODDEN CROSS HANGING ON THE WALL BY THE ENTRANCE OF THE FLAT, WAS MIRACOUSLY LIKE PROJECTED TOWARDS ME, ALMOST AS DETACHING ITSELF FROM THE WALL. IT REMAINED AS HANGING IN THE AIR PERHAPS FOR 1 OR 2 SECONDS FACING ME!!!

I MUST SAY IT WAS ASTONISHING AND EXCATLY WHAT I REALY NEEDED TOO!!!

ONE MORE TIME I COUNSELLED MYSELF, EMBRACING THE CROSS AND POURING ON IT ALL MY ANGER, BITTERNESS AND MORE, ALLOWING THE CROSS AND/BLOOD OF OUR SAVIOUR TO SWALLOW AND ABSORBE ALL THIS TOXINE THAT WAS POISONING ME WITHIN. ONLY THEN I WAS ABLE TO FIND PEACE AGAIN WITH GOD, MYSELF, AND THIS MAN TOO.

YOU CAN CERTAINLY RECALL THE LORD JESUS CREATING A LINK AND A COMPARISON WITH HIS SACRIFICE AND THE

LIFTING UP OF THE SERPENT BY MOSES IN THE WILDERNESS WANDERING IN NUM 21:9, WHICH SAYS: < SO MOSES MADE A BRONZE SERPENT, AND PUIT IT ON A POLE; AND SO IT WAS, IF A SERPENT HAD BITTEN ANYONE, WHEN HE LOOKED AT THE BRONZE SERPENT, HE LIVED. > CF. ALSO JOHN 3: 14-16.

I THINK IT IS WONDERFUL THAT HE IS OUR VICTORY AND OUR SOLUTION, AND THAT HIS SCRIPTURES HELP US TO UNDERSTAND AND TO DEAL WITH OUR EXPERIENCES.

TO SATISFY YOUR CURIOUSITY, DO KNOW THAT ALL CAME TO NOTHING AS FIRST THIS PERSON CUT ME OFF COMPLETELY FROM ANY POSSIBILITY TO RECIEVE COMMISSIONS FROM HIS SIDE, AND SECONDLY THE DEAL FAILED TOTALLY, AS WITHOUT DOUBT THIS WAS A FAKED REFINERY JUST TRYING TO STEAL MONEY FROM INEXPERIENCED BUYERS, WTH THE EXCUSE OF ASKING FOR A CONTRACT REGISTRATION FEE. IN CONCLUSION, FOR THIS AND OTHER REASONS SUCH AS KNOWING A COLLEGUE IN MINISTRY TOO WHO THOUGH HAVING HELPED SELLING REAL DIAMONDS SEVEN TIMES AND NEVER GOT PAYED, I DO NOT PURSUE THIS KIND OF BUSINESS ANY LONGER, BUT I FOCUS ON GOD'S WORK AND CALLING ON MY LIFE; NEITHER DO I WANT TO BE AN ACTIVE PART OF ANY COMPANY THAT WOULD GUARANTEE ME ANY COMMISSIONS. SADLY EVEN TODAY, AND PERHAPS MORE THAN IN THE PAST TOO, WE ARE TO BEWARE OF WOLVES IN SHEEP CLOTHES AND BE MORE DISCERNING THROUGH HIS GRACE AS THE LORD TELLS US IN LUKE 10:3: < "GO YOUR WAY; BEHOLD, I SEND YOU OUT AS LAMBS

AMONG WOLVES. > PLEASE SEE ALSO JOHN 10:12.

****

THE NEXT EPISODE I WOULD LIKE TO TELL YOU ABOUT HAS
ALSO AN ATTRACTION AND BEAUTY OF ITS OWN. WE ARE
GOING BACK AGAIN TO TWELVE OR FORTEEN YEARS AGO',
AND I MAY HAVE BEEN STILL IN BIBLE COLLEGE THEN.

I RECALL THAT I WAS WORKING IN THAT PREVIOUSLY
MENTIONED RESTAURANT IN PICCADILLY, WHICH WAS
CERTAINLY A BLESSING AS IT HAD HELPED ME TO FINANCE
MY STUDIES FOR THE MINISTRY FOR MANY YEARS. IN FACT
IT WAS AND STILL IS AN EXCLUSIVE AND ATTRACTIVE PLACE
TO WORK IN; AND I WORKED THERE ALSO FOR ONE YEAR IN
88-89. BY THE WAY, AMONG MANY OTHER INTERESTING
PEOPLE, IT WAS IN THIS YEAR I THINK THAT I MUST HAVE
SERVED ONE OF THE HASBAND OF MARYLINE MONROE ',
THAT IS: ARTHUR MILLER, THE FAMOUS SCREEN WRITER.
ONCE I REMEMBER WHEN SERVING HIM SOME NEW
POTATOES, HE HAD ASKED ME FOR ONLY ONE, AND
HAVING REPLIED TO HIM "WHICH ONE? ", HE LAUGHED.

ANYHOW IT HAPPENED THAT IN 1995 I HAD COME BACK TO
WORK IN THIS RESTAURANT ALSO THROUGH THE HELP OF
THE MANAGERESS THERE ALREADY KNOWN TO ME FROM

1989. IT IS PERHAPS COMMON THAT IN ALL WORK PLACES WE HAVE DISAGREEMENTS AND FRICTIONS, AS ALSO WE HAD SOMETIMES HERE TOO.

I MUST CONFESS THAT I AND AN OTHER MANAGER WERE NOT IN VERY CLOSE TERMS, ALTHOUGH I WAS TRYING TO KEEP IN PEACE WITH ALL; BUT LIFE IS LIKE THIS AFTER ALL. STILL I DO NOT KNOW IF HE WAS A BIT JELOUS..., BUT I DO KNOW THAT HE MUST HAVE HELD RATHER A RESTRICTED VIEW OF CHRISTIANITY, AS IN FACT ONCE HE HAD ASKED ME NOT A VERY NICE QUESTION AT ALL REGARDING OUR CHURCH. BUT NEVERMIND, AND APART FOR TOO MANY SCREAMS WE WERE NOT TOO BAD AFTER ALL. ONE EVENING HOWEVER, I BELIEVE DURING THE BUSY CHRISTMAS PERIOD WE DID HAVE A DISAGREEMENT IN OUR WORK AND I HAD MADE A COMPLAIN TO MY OTHER MANAGER AS TO WHAT HE HAD DONE REGARDING OUR SERVICE PREPARATION.

WELL HAVING HEARD ABOUT IT, I SUDDENLY SAW HIM COMING TOWARDS ME SHOUTING AT ME AND PHYSICALLY PUSHING ME WITH HIS HANDS ON MY CHEST.

BEING A VERY SENSITIVE PERSON I CERTAINLY WAS NOT HAPPY ABOUT IT.

I DO NOT REMEMBER EXCATLY WHAT HAPENED NEXT WHETHER HE DID APOLOGISE OR NOT. HOWEVER A FEW DAYS AFTER I TOLD THEM THAT I HAD REPORTED THIS TO THE POLICE AS A WARNING, THOUGH WITHOUT SPECIFYING THE NAME OF THE PERSON; VERY CLEARLY THE POLICE

OFFICER ASSURED ME THAT IF ANY FURTHER PROBLEM TO LET THEM KNOW AS I HAD THE RIGHT TO WORK THERE WITHOUT ANYBODY TOUCHING ME WITH A FINGER. THOUGH I WAS QUITE CONFIDENT ABOUT MY JOB POSITION AND ALSO I KNEW THAT I WAS ON THE RIGHT SIDE AS I ONLY HAD COMPLAINED FOR THE WELL BEING OF THE SERVICE IN THE RESTAURANT, I MUST SAY THAT I WAS FEELING RATHER DOWN BECASUSE OF THE OFFENCE AND BEING AWARE THAT THE MANAGERS WERE QUITE CLOSE TO ONE ANOTHER IN MUTUAL SUPPORT TOO; IN FACT SOME TIME LATER, ANOTHER ONE, WITH AN EXCUSE, PUSHED ME TOO.

NEVERMIND; SO IT HAPPENED THAT ONE EVENING AFTER THIS ACCIDENT, OR INDEED THE SAME EVENING, I WAS JUST STRUGGLING TO REST AT NIGHT AND I WAS RATHER EMOTIONAL TOO, BEING AFFECTIONATE TO THIS WORK PLACE TOO.

SUDDENLY SOMETHING WONDERFUL STARTED TO HAPPEN WHILE LYING IN BED. RIGHT THERE, INSIDE MY SHEETS, I STARTED TO HEAR A BEAUTIFUL MUSICAL TUNE AND WORDS OF WORSHIP TOWARDS GOD; STRAIGHT AWAY IT BEGAN TO OVERWHELM ME AND MY EMOTIONS, FILLING ALL MY ENVIROMENT. I WAS SOAKING AGAIN IN HIS PRESENCE! ONCE AGAIN HE WAS HEALING ME WITH THE CONFORT OF HIS WINGS AS IN MAL. 4:2 < BUT TO YOU WHO FEAR MY NAME THE SUN OF RIGHTEOUSNESS SHALL ARISE WITH HEALING IN HIS WINGS; AND YOU SHALL GO OUT AND GROW FAT AS STALL-FED CALVES. > I SAY AMEN

TO THIS.

I STILL REMEMBER AND I AM NOT SURPRISED EITHER THAT THE SONG WAS ONE OF OUR FAVOURATE IN OUR CHURCH SERVICES TOO.

FROM THE SCRIPTURES I LEARNED THAT HE WAS THE LORD JESUS THAT WAS PRAISING GOD IN MY PRESENCE [HEBR. 2:12], AND ALSO CONFORTING ME SO TO ENABLE ME TO BETTER CONFORT OTHERS! HERE WE ARE ENCOURAGED BY 2 COR. 1:4 < WHO CONFORTS US IN ALL OUR TRIBULATION, THAT WE MAY BE ABLE TO CONFORT THOSE WHO ARE IN ANY TROUBLE, WITH THE CONFORT WITH WHICH WE OURSELVES ARE CONFORTED BY GOD. >

AFTER THIS, FEELING CLOSER TO HIM AND MORE IN ONE PIECE THAN BEFORE, MY LIFE AT WORK CARRIED ON AS USUAL WITH NO MORE OF THIS KIND OF PROBLEMS.

I HOPE AND TO HIS GLORY THAT THIS HAS SOMEHOW MINISTERED TO YOU TOO, AS IT IS ALWAYS ABOUT HIS SAVING GRACE AND NOT OUR HUMAN/RELIGIOUS ATTEMPTS TO RIGHTEOUSNESS AND WORKS, AS IT IS FOR EXAMPLE ACCORDING SOME OTHER BELIEFS!

****

AT THIS POINT I WOULD LIKE TO MOVE ON AND TELL YOU OF, I BELIEVE AN OTHER AFFASCINATING EXPERIENCE THAT I HAD TOWARDS THE END OF MY BIBLE COLLEGE IN 1999. IT

WAS TOWARDS THE END OF THE COURSE I THINK, THAT EACH STUDENT OF THE SECOND YEAR OF IBIOL [THE HIGHER DIPLOMA OF CHRISTIAN MINISTRY], WAS ASKED TO PREPARE A LITTLE 20 MINUTES SERMON, I THINK FROM THE PASTORAL EPISTLES. I BILIEVE TO HAVE CHOSEN 1 TIMOTHY 4 FROM V. 1 TO MAYBE V. 3-5.

JUST TO GIVE YOU A SMALL BACKGROUND FOR WHAT FOLLOWS, IN THOSE DAYS I WAS SOMETIMES SOCIALISING WITH A SON OF A COLONNEL AND THEN MADE GENERAL, I THINK KILLED OR JUST DEAD ANYWAY, A WIDOW OF AN OTHER GENERAL, AND AN OTHER WOMAN DESCENDENT FROM A FAMILY OF GENERALS, AND PERHAPS EVEN OF ROYAL BOOD TOO. BY THE WAY THEY ALL CAME AS GUESTS FOR MY GRADUATION SERVICE.

NOW HERE WE WERE IN THE CLASS, ME AND THE OTHER STUDENTS, EACH WAITING TO BE CALLED TO GIVE HIS LITTLE SERMON. I AM CONVINCED STILL THAT WHAT I GAVE THEM WAS A GOOD PROPHETIC MESSAGE. PLEASE DO EMBRACE YOURSELF AS I NEED TO NARRATE IT HERE FOR YOU TOO AS PART OF WHAT HAPPENED. PLEASE KEEP IN MIND THAT I HAD JUST QUICKLY PREPARED A SKELETON OF IT WITHOUT MUCH PREPARATION, ALSO BECAUSE OF MY RATHER BUSY DAYS. HOWEVER IN MY SPIRIT I KNEW THAT IT WAS JUST THE SERMON WHICH I WANTED TO PREACH.

NOW FOR VARIOUS REASONS I SHALL BE EXPOSING JUST THE MAIN PART OF IT, IF I MAY SAY THIS. SO MY TURN CAME, AND THERE I WAS STANDING IN FRONT OF THE OTHER STUDENTS AND SOMEONE POINTING A BIG CAMERA

ON ME LIKE IN A FILM. I WAS ABOUT TO DELIVER MY FIRST EVER SERMON. PLEASE DO NOTE THAT THERE MAY BE SOME VERY FEW AND TINY CHANGES. SO IF YOU ARE READY, HERE WE GO!

AS ALREADY MENTIONED I PREACHED FROM 1 TIM. 4: 1FF, WHICH PARTIALLY SAYS < NOW THE SPIRIT EXPRESSELY SAYS THAT IN LATTER TIMES SOME WILL DEPART FROM THE FAITH, GIVING HEED TO DECIEVING SPIRITS AND DOCTRINES OF DEMONS, SPEAKING LIES IN HYPOCRISY, HAVING THEIR OWN CONSCIENCE SEARED WITH A HOT IRON,...>

AND SO I AM STARTING: < ....ABOUT 5 YEARS AGO' DURING MY JOURNEY, I ENTERED INTO THE CITY OF BABYLON. BABYLON WAS VERY BEAUTIFUL, HER NECK WAS ADORNED WITH THICK AND HEAVY PURE GOLDEN CHAINS; GOLDEN RINGS AND A LARGE PURE DIAMOND RING WERE ON HER FINGERS. HER UNCLE HAD BEEN HIGH PRIEST ALSO IN CHARGE OF THE WEEKLY PRAYERS WITH THE KING. AND THOUGH A CHRISTIAN, IN THOSE DAYS I WAS WORSHIPPING THE BEAST! BABYLON HAD BEAUTIFUL TOWERS [BRESTS]. BUT A DEEP SCAR WAS RUNNING OVER THEM FROM ONE END TO AN OTHER. SO SHE COVERED THE SCAR WITH A BEAUTIFUL PAINTING OF PINK FLOWERS, AND THE NATIONS KEPT DRINKING FROM THE MADDENING MILK AND WINE OF HER ADULTERIES. AND I ALSO SINNED AGAINST GOD!

IN THE SAME WEEK, BABYLON WAS ENTHRONED QUEEN OF

HEAVEN, HER HEAD WAS CRUSHED IN A CAR ACCIDENT, AND A CROWN OF METAL STAPLES FROM ONE END TO AN OTHER, WAS PLACED UPON HER HEAD TO HOLD IT TOGETHER! ALSO HER PROUD CHIN WAS CRUSHED AND REPLACED WITH A PLASTIC ONE...>.

AS ALREADY MENTIONED ABOVE I ALSO ADDED OTHER THINGS IN MY MESSAGE. AT ABOUT IN THE MIDDLE OF THIS, SUDDENLY THE SPIRIT OF THE LORD FELL ON ME; REALLY IT STARTED TO FIGHT AGAINST ME, LIKE EMBRACING ME AND PULLING AND PUSHING ME BACK AND FORWARD, AND LEFT AND RIGHT. PLEASE DO KNOW THAT I WAS ALMOST FEELING AS BEING OVERPOWERED AT ANY MOMENT BY HIM BENDING ME, TO A POINT EVEN NOT TOO FAR FROM TOUCHING THE GROUND! IT WAS A REAL PHISICAL FIGHT MAYBE LIKE JACOB HAD [GEN. 32:22-24]. BY THE WAY I UNDERSTOOD THIS LAST LINK, ONLY MANY MONTHS AFTERWARDS. ANYHOW THE FIGHT STOPPED WHEN IN A CERTAIN MOMENT, REMEMBERING HIS WORD OF ENCOURAGEMENT TO ME IN AN OTHER EXPERIENCE, I MANAGED TO SHAKE HIM OFF, IF I MAY ARE DO SAY SO. THUS I WAS ABLE TO STAND STRAIGHT AND CONTINUE TO DELIVER THE MESSAGE TILL THE END, SEEING ALSO MY COLLEGUES STUDENTS LOOKING RATHER PERPLEXED.

WELL I WAS TOLD THAT THIS MESSAGE HAD BEEN A BLESSING TO THEM, AND I HOPE THIS WAS A BLESSING TO YOU TOO. IN FACT THERE HAD BEEN SOME IDOLATROUS ASPECTS IN MY FRIENDSHIP WITH THIS PERSON ABOVE; BUT GOD HAD TOLD ME OFF IN HIS MERCY; BY HIS GRACE ALSO SHE WAS CONVINCED BY ME TO COME TO CHURCH A

FEW TIMES. INDEED THE BIBLE MAKES IT CLEAR THAT WE MUST COME APART FROM ANY IDOLS, AND ANY KIND OF IDOLATRY IS ULTIMATELY DIRECTED TO THE DEVIL [2 COR. 6:11-18; REV.17-19]. AND AS YOU KNOW BOTH OUR WORDS AND BEHAVIOUR NEEDS TO REMAIN BOTH LED AND JUSTIFIED BY THE SCRIPTURES; IN THIS AND IN THE SPIRIT OF THE LORD IS OUR STRENGTH.

HOWEVER THIS DID NOT END JUST HERE.

DO KNOW THAT DURING MY SERMON I HAD THE BURDEN TO SAY SOMETHING REGARDING A PASTOR, BUT I DID NOT DO THIS DESPITE THE BURDEN WHICH WAS ON ME, THAT I NOW AM CONVINCED WAS FROM GOD. THEN IT FOLLOWED THAT, I BELIEVE THE DAY AFTER, WE WERE IN THE CLASS AS USUAL; NOW THE TIME FOR THE BREAK CAME, AND I STILL REMEMBER THAT I WAS HAVING A LITTLE DRINK WHEN A FEMALE STUDENT FROM ASIA APPROACHED ME TELLING ME THAT SHE HAD A MESSAGE FROM THE HOLY SPIRIT.

I DID SAY OK TO HER AND BOWED MY BACK AND MY HEAD TO HER, TO HEAR WHAT SHE HAD TO SAY. INTERESTINGLY SHE STOOD BEHIND ME AND SHE BEGAN TO HIT ME HARD ON MY BACK WITH HER BEAR HANDS! SHE KEPT DOING THIS FOR ABOUT 5 MINUTES I THINK, AT THE SAME TIME SHE WAS TELLING ME THAT I HAD TO SAY WHAT THE HOLY SPIRIT WANTED ME TO SAY, AND I HAD NOT OBEYED HIM [THAT IS THE DAY BEFORE]. BASICALLY AT SOME BRIEF INTERVALS SHE WOULD SMACK ME HARD, THE SHE WOULD TELL ME TO OBEY THE HOLY SPIRIT WHEN I HAVE TO SAY

SOMETHING, AND ALSO THAT GOD LOVED ME VERY MUCH.
ONCE AGAIN I MUST THANK GOD FOR THAT STRONG
REBUKE! AS WE ARE TO LOVE THE DISCIPLINE OF THE LORD
[HEBR. 12:1-11].

THIS IS VERY IMPORTANT, BEING IN OUR SINFUL NATURE
WE HAVE OFTEN THE TENDENCY TO BE ARROGANT, PROUD
AND STIFF-NECKED AS IN 2 CHRON. 30:8 < "DO NOT
BE STIFF-NECKED AS YOUR FATHERS WERE; BUT YELD
YOURSELVES TO THE LORD; AND ENTER HIS SANCTUARY,
WHICH HE HAS SANTIFIED FOREVER, AND SERVE THE LORD
YOUR GOD, THAT THE FIERCENESS OF HIS WRATH MAY
TURN AWAY FROM YOU. >

THOUGH I KNOW THAT YOU KNOW WHAT I AM TALKING
ABOUT, I JUST WANT TO GIVE YOU TWO VERY BRIEFS
EXAMPLES TO FURTHER ILLUSTRATE THIS POINT, AND BY
THE WAY HIS REBUKES ARE MANY MORE IN MY LIFE
UNFORTUNATELY. FOR EXAMPLE I CAN RECALL ONCE TO BE
LOOKING AT MYSELF IN THE MIRROW OF A TOILETTE,
FEELING RATHER STUPID/ARROGANT. SUDDENLY AS I BENT
MY HEAD TO WASH MY HANDS AND FACE, THE LORD
BROUGHT IT DOWN A LITTLE BIT FURTHER IN ORDER THAT I
MYSELF BANGED HARD MY HEAD TO THE MARBLE OF THE
SINK RATHER PAINFULLY TOO; THEN SUDDENLY I FELT AS
SOMEONE BEHIND ME HAD JUST TOUCHED WITH HIS
HANDS MY SHOULDER, MAKING ME FEEL THAT HE WAS
RECONFIRMING HIS LOVE TO ME. WHAT WAS ALSO
ASTONISHING IS THAT NO MARK WAS LEFT ON MY

FORHEAD.

IN AN OTHER OCCASION I REMEMBER BEING IN THE UNDERGROUND WAITING FOR THE TRAIN. THERE AGAIN I BELIEVE I WAS FEELING STILL ARROGANT AND TOO PROUD; SUDDENLY THE SPIRIT OF THE LORD LIFTED MY LEG MORE THAN I HAD INTENDED IT TO REACH AS I WAS APPROACCHING THE ARRIVING TRAIN. I WAS STILL TOO FAR FROM THE TRAIN AND NOTHING HAPPENED; BUT I MUST CONFESS THAT I WAS A BIT SHOCKED AND SCARED. I THOUGHT THE MEANING OF IT TO BE QUITE CLEAR TO ME: I TOOK IT AS HE MEANT SOMETHING LIKE THIS: HE IS EVERYTHING AND I AM NOTHING WITHOUT HIM AND COMPARED TO HIM; ALSO BEING LORD OVER MY LIFE HE CAN ALSO KILL ME AT ANY TIME IF HE WANTS TOO, BECAUSE OUR LOVING FATHER IS ALSO CONSUMING FIRE, AND SHOWS NO PARTIALITY TO NOONE [1 COR. 10:1-13].

GOING BACK TO OUR MAIN STORY, FOR YOU OWN CURIOUSITY, DO KNOW THAT FOR A FEW DAYS I HAD CLEAR RED MARKS ON MY BACK; FUNNILY, A FEW DAYS AFTER THIS INCIDENT HAPPENED [THE BEATING], THIS SAME WOMAN CAME TO ME , IN A WAY EXCUSING HERSELF SAYING THAT SHE WAS STILL LEARNING HOW TO GIVE MESSAGES TO PEOPLE IN A CONTROLLED MANNER, PERHAPS ALLUDING TO 1 COR.14:31-32: < FOR YOU CAN ALL PROPHESY ONE BY ONE, THAT ALL MAY LEARN AND THAT ALL MAY BE ENCOURAGED. AND THE SPIRITS OF THE PROPHETS ARE SUBJECT TO THE PROPHETS. >

WELL WHATEVER WAY GOD WANTED TO REBUKE ME FOR,

BLESS HIS HOLY NAME ANYWAY!

****

THE EPISODE THAT FOLLOWS NEXT HAS SOME INTERESTING
ASPECTS WITHOUT DOUBT, THAT I BELIEVE WILL BE A
BLESSING TO MANY, DESPITE IT CERTAINLY HAS AN UGLY
SIDE TO IT. SADLY VERY HUMAN AND REALISTIC TO THE
WORLD IN WHICH WE LIVE.

AS I HAVE ALREADY MENTIONED TO YOU IN THE
INTRODUCTION, IN MY YEARS AS A YOUNG MAN, I
SUFFERED A LOT OF SPIRITUAL DEPRESSION AND FOR LONG
TIME TOO, MAINLY DUE TO THE FACT THAT THE DEVIL WAS
TAKING ADVANTAGE OF MY SPIRITUAL IGNORANCE,
BACKSLIDENESS, AND ESPECIALLY KNOWING THAT I HAD A
CALLING FROM GOD TOWARDS THE MINISTRY! AND SO
THIS KIND OF SITUATION CONTINUED IN LONDON TOO FOR
SOME YEARS; ALSO LIVING HERE WITHOUT A FAMILY HAD
ITS OWN DISADVANTAGES. SO FOR THE ABOVE
MENTIONED REASONS, ESPECIALLY IN THE EIGHTIES I WAS
OFTEN PARTAKING IN SEXUAL IMMORALITY. I DO NOT NEED
TO TELL YOU THE CONSEQUENCES AS YOU CAN MOSTLY
IMMAGINE YOURSELF; HOWEVER USUALLY PEOPLE
ENSLAVED BY THIS SINFUL HABIT, WOULD SUFFER
DEMONIC INFLUENCE AND ITS CONSEQUENCES, LOSS OF
SELF DIGNITY, VALUE, PURITY, HOLINESS, GOD'S AND
MAN'S FAVOUR, LOSS OF TIME IN BUILDING THE PRESENT

AND THE FUTURE, ENERGY, SLEEP, AND FINANCIAL RESOURCES, AND LOSS OF GENERAL HEALTH, EVEN AT TIMES CATCHING DESEASES TOO; AND LET US NOT TALK ABOUT UNWANTED PREGNANCIES, ABORTIONS, FAMILY'S PROBLEMS LINKED COSTLY SOCIAL AND COMMUNITY ISSUES.

ANYHOW GRADUALLY THE LORD WAS ALSO TAKING ME THROUGH A PROCESS OF SANTIFICATION FOR SOME YEARS, AND FINALLY IN 93 FILLED ME WITH THE HOLY SPIRIT, AN EXPERIENCE THAT CHANGED ME DRAMMATICALLY EVEN MORE, ENABLING ME TO SOON TO BE TOTALLY COMMITTED TO HIM, EVEN SHARING IN HIS GLORY AND DOING HIS ORDAINED WORK.

WELL IT HAPPENED THAT IN 94 I WAS SOMETIMES ALSO SOCIALISING WITH A WOMAN FROM A NOBLE AND RICH FAMILY; AND AT TIMES SHE WAS LONELY AND SUFFERED FROM DEPRESSION. PLEASE REMEMBER THAT JESUS CAME TO GIVE US LIFE TO THE FULNESS AS WE SEE IN JOHN 10:10 < "THE THIEF DOES NOT COME EXCEPT TO STEAL, AND TO KILL AND TO DESTROY. I HAVE COME THAT THEY MAY HAVE LIFE, AND THAT THEY MAY HAVE IT MORE ABUNDANTLY. >

NOTE THAT I MYSELF FOR MANY YEARS I HAVE NOT BEEN SUFFERING THAT KIND OF DEPRESSION ANY LONGER; INTERESTINGLY ALSO IN MY CASE THIS CHANGE GRADUALLY HAPPENED WITHOUT THE NEED OF MEDICATION, AND IT IS THE GRACE OF GOD THAT HELPS ME TO MANTAIN A BALANCED LIFE IN THE MIDST OF OUR HUMAN DIFFICULTIES. THOUGH AS ALREADY MENTIONED I DO AM

AWARE THAT AT TIMES THESE MEDICATIONS ARE
NECESSARY, I ALSO BELIEVE THAT THERE IS A GREAT ABUSE
IN THE USE OF PILLS, AND ALL THIS CONTEXT IS MADE EVEN
MORE SENSITIVE AND COMPLEX DUE TO THE FINANCIAL
SIDE OF IT. IN FACT IN THE WORDS OF A PSYCHIATRIC
WHOM I MET A FEW DAYS AGO', IT SEEMS THAT THIS
MEDICAL CARE IS SOMEHOW RATHER STIMULATED AND
ORIENTATED BY AND AROUND THE BUSINESS SIDE OF IT!

WELL THIS LADY ALSO HAD A WEAKNESS
TOWARDS SEXUAL IMMORALITY, MUCH SPIRITUAL
IGNORANCE, AND EVEN TODAY I DO NOT KNOW WHERE
SHE STANDS IN HER RELATIONSHIP WITH GOD.

ANYHOW, I WAS HOPING THAT SHE WOULD GET BETTER,
AND BEING MUCH YOUNGER AND LESS EXPERIENCED, BY
THE WAY I CERTAINLY DO NOT SOCIALISE WITH HER
ANYMORE NOW, I WENT TO VISIT HER TO TAKE HER
OUT FOR A COFFE .

THERE I WAS WAITING FOR HER IN THE SITTING ROOM OF
HER FLAT WAITING FOR HER AS SHE WAS GETTING
CHANGED IN HER BEDROOM. SUDDENLY SHE STARTED TO
CALL ME AND INVITE ME TO GO TO HER BEDROOM. AFTER
REFUSING A FEW TIMES EXPLAINING TO HER THAT I WOULD
PREFER TO WAIT THERE WHERE I WAS, SHE ASKED ME
AGAIN TO GO TO HER BEDROOM INFORMING ME ALSO
THAT SHE HAD £5,OOO IN HER BEDSIDE TABLE! SO
I CONTINUED TO PRAY, [A GOOD IDEA FOR A YOUNG
CHRISTIAN MAN IN THOSE OCCASIONS IN PARTICULAR],
AND AS SOON AS I REFUSED AGAIN AND TOLD HER TO

HURRY UP SO THAT WE COULD GO OUT; SUDDENLY INSIDE MY BOSOM I FELT AS SOMEONE WAS JUMPING UP AND DOWN OF JOY!!!

IT WAS LIKE A LIVING PERSON MOVING POWERFULLY AND INTENSELY WITHIN ME; PERHAPS NOT EXCATLY AS A PREGNANT PERSON OF COURSE, BUT SOMEHOW SIMILARLY, AS BELIEVERS ARE REALLY PREAGNANT WITH THE HOLY SPIRIT. IT WAS WONDERFUL, AND STILL TODAY I THINK THAT IT WAS THE HOLY SPIRIT WITHIN ME WHO WAS REJOICING IN MY DECISION OF OBEDIENCE AND FAITHFULNESS TO HIM, WITH A CLEAR AND PRACTICAL PROOF THAT I LOVED HIM AND I WANTED TO OBEY HIS COMMANDMENTS, AS ONLY THIS IS THE TRUE LOVE WHICH CAN ALLOW THE FATHER AND THE SON TO MAKE THEIR HOME IN US, AS WE CAN SEE IN JOHN 14:23: < JESUS ANSWERED AND SAID TO HIM, "IF ANYONE LOVES ME, HE WILL KEEP MY WORD; AND MY FATHER WILL LOVE HIM, AND WE WILL COME TO HIM AND MAKE OUR HOME WITH HIM. >

TO GOD'S GLORY, I THEN TOOK HER OUT WITHOUT ANY OF US SUFFERING ANY HARM.

IN TIME AHEAD I REALISED THAT HER MENTALITY WAS DIFFERENT, AND SO I DISTANCED MYSELF AND SOON I STOPPED SOCIALISING WITH HER COMPLETELY. IT IS IMPORTANT TO KEEP IN MIND THAT BAD COMPANY CORRUPTS GOOD CHARACTER [1COR. 5:6-7], AND WE MUST ALSO DISCERN AND BE AWARE OF THE FACT THAT UNFOUTUNATELY SOME MAY DO A LITTLE OF THE

CHRISTIAN TALK, BUT NOT REALLY DO THE WALK; THESE MAY BE THE PEOPLE THAT REFLECT RELIGION MORE THAN A PERSONAL RELATIONSHIP WITH THE LORD JESUS OF NAZARETH! [MATTH.7:21-23].

****

TOWARDS THE END OF THIS CHAPTER HERE IS ANOTHER SMALL STORY WHICH ALSO IS VERY RECENT, TO BE PRECISE THIS EASTER ON THE 24TH-APRIL-2011; FOR I DO NOT WISH TO BOTHER YOU BY TELLING YOU OF AT LEAST 2 TIMES WHEN I FELT ALMOST AS BEING TRANSFIGURED AND PEOPLE IN FRONT ME WERE STARING AT ME IN AMESAMENT AT THE SURROUNDING PRESENCE OF GOD; NEITHER DO I WISH TO BOTHER YOU BY TELLING YOU THAT AT LEAST IN TWO OCCASIONS DURING THE WORSHIP I FELT AS THE HOLY SPIRIT STRETCHED MY PHYSICAL BODY FOR 2-3 SECONDS BEJOND MY NATURAL HEIGHT CAUSING ME TO LOOK TALLER THAN OTHER PEOPLE AROUND ME WHO WERE REALLY PHSYCALLY TALLER THAN ME, AT THE AMEZEMENT OF PEOPLE AROUND ME, SUCH AS ONCE IN THE BIBLE COLLEGE. AND THOUGH I BELIEVE I AM SAYING THE TRUTH, I WOULD NOT BE ABLE TO PROVE THESE LAST TWO EXPERIENCES FROM THE SCRIPTURES, EXCEPT FOR THE FACT THAT ONLY THE LORD JESUS CHRIST WAS SEEN TRANSFIGURED; AND THEREFORE I WOULD NEITHER EXPECT YOU TO BELIEVE THEM TOO; BUT PLEASE DO

FORGIVE ME AS FOR SOME REASONS I NEEDED TO MENTIONED THEM VERY BRIEFLY HERE IN THIS WAY.

NOW AS I CONTINUE TO WRITE THIS BOOK TODAY IS IN FACT THE 9TH OF MAY 2011, AND EASTER SUNDAY WAS JUST TWO WEEKS AGO'.

IN THE AFTERNOON I HAD DECIDED TO TAKE A BRAKE FROM OUR SMALL PRAYER MEETING AND SO, KNOWING THAT I HAD THE TIME TO PAY A VISIT TO THE PATIENTS OF A PSHYCHIATRIC HOSPITAL NOT FAR FROM MY CHURCH, AT ABOUT THREE IN THE AFTERNOON I MADE MY WAY TOWARDS IT [I HAVE ALREADY MENTIONED TO YOU THAT I HAVE FAIRLY REGULARLY MADE THESE VISITS ALREADY FOR THE LAST 14 YEARS]. IN MY WAY THERE, AS USUALLY I BEGAN TO PRAY FOR GOD'S GRACE AND FAVOUR, AND OBVIOULSLY FOR DIVINE APPOINTMENTS TO DO HIS WORK ACCORDING TO HIS WILL. AT THE RECEPTION THEY ARE ALWAYS KIND AND LET ME IN ONCE I TELL THEM THAT I AM A CHURCH PASTOR WITH THE DESIRE TO SPEND SOME TIME WITH PATIENTS, PRAYING WITH THEM, HELP/CHAT WITH THEM, AND EVEN HAVE BIBLE READING AND DISCUSSIONS WITH WHOEVER WANTS TO.

ANYHOW HAVING ENTERED IN THE WARD I INFORMED THE STAFF AND SOME PATIENTS AROUND THAT I WAS GOING TO BE IN THE SITTING ROOM BEING AVAILABLE FOR THEM, WOULD ANYONE LIKE TO SEE ME. TO MY SURPRISE AND GLADNESS ON TV WAS ON THE MUSICAL "MARY POPPINS ",

AND SOME PATIENTS WERE WATCHING IT.

YOU MAY BE SURPRISED BUT I GO THERE ALSO TO ENJOY
MYSELF, THOUGH I DO NOT LIKE TO BE LOCKED IN
WITH THEM! AND SINCE KINGDOM LIFE IS LIFE IN
ABUNDANCE, THE LORD NEVER LETS ME DOWN AS ALWAYS
PROVIDES SOME EXCITEMENT FOR ME. SO ONCE
I INTRODUCED MYSELF I STARTED TO WATCH THE MUSICAL
GLADLY, ESPECIALLY AS I DO NOT KEEP A TV WHERE I LIVE. I
THEN BEGAN TO TALK WITH AN EGYPTIAN PATIENT, WHO
AFTER KNOWING THAT I WAS ITALIAN, HE EXPRESSED HIS
DESIRE TO ME THAT HE WAS LOOKING FOR AN ITALIAN
WIFE. ON MY RIGHT THERE WAS ALSO AN ELDER LADY
FROM BANGLADESH WHO WAS INTERESTED TO PRAY AND
TALK WITH ME. WE DID EXCHANGE A FEW WORDS THOUGH
SHE COULD HARDLY SPEAK ENGLISH, BUT WHEN SHE
REALISED THAT I WAS MORE INTERESTED TO WATCH THE
TV, AS I REALLY NEEDED A BREAK AND IT WAS EASTER ALSO
FOR ME, SHE GOT UP LOOKING ANGRY AGAINST ME AND
LEFT THE ROOM.

WELL THE MUSICAL WAS AMUSING I MUST SAY, AND FOR A
CHANGE, NO SCENES OF VIOLENCE NOR PORNOGRAPHY
WERE SHOWN; SOON IT ENDED AND I, FEELING MORE
RESTED I CONTINUED TO TALK WITH PATIENTS THERE. IN
MY CONVERSATION WITH THE EGIPTIAN GENTLEMAN,
WHO WAS ALSO A CHRISTIAN CATHOLIC, I WAS POINTING
OUT TO HIM THE PRIORITY TO DO GOD'S KINGDOM WORK
FIRST; ALSO THE NEED TO GIVE LESS IMPORTANCE TO THE
DESIRE TO MARRY, ASSURING HIM THAT IT IS GOD'S
PROMISE TO PROVIDE FOR US EVERY THING THAT WE NEED

ONCE WE SEEK HIS KINGDOM FIRST AS IN MATTH. 6:25-34: <...."BUT SEEK FIRST THE KINGDOM OF GOD AND HIS RIGHTEOUSNESS, AND ALL THESE THINGS SHALL BE ADDED TO YOU... >

INTERESTING, AND I BELIEVE IN ANSWER TO MY PRAYERS, THE LADY FROM BANGLADESH HAD COME BACK AND WAS SITTING OPPOSITE US LISTENING, AS WE WERE HAVING OUR CONVERSATION. AT A CERTAIN POINT THE MAN, WITHOUT GIVING ME TIME TO PRAY AS WE HAD PREVIOUSLY AGREED, GOT UP, GREETED ME AND LEFT [I DID MANAGE TO INVITE HIM TO OUR CHURCH BY THE WAY, AS A BIT MORE OF SINGING WILL DO HIM WELL]. THEN I STARTED AGAIN TO SPEAK WITH THE LADY. ONCE SHE SAT CLOSE TO ME, SHE APOLOGIZED FOR HER BAD ENGLISH; I DO NOT KNOW WHY BUT IN HER MOUTH THERE WAS A LOT OF SALIVA POSSIBLY BECAUSE OF WHAT SHE WAS CHEWING. I COULD SEE THAT SHE WAS FROM A GOOD FAMILY AND HAD A GOOD HEART; I EXPLAINED TO HER THE WORK AND THE GRACE OF OUR LORD JESUS, AND TO MY GREAT JOY SHE ASK ME TO PRAY THE LORD'S PRAYER WITH ME AS IT IS IN ROM 10.

SLOWLY AND WITH A FEW REPETITIONS, I LED HER IN THE LORD'S PRAYER, AS SHE ACCEPTED THE LORD JESUS AS HER PERSONAL LORD AND SAVIOUR. THEN SHE LOOKED HAPPY AND THANKED ME, AND TO MY AMAZEMENT STRAIGHTAWAY THE NURSE CAME TELLING HER THAT HER FAMILY WAS HERE TO VISIT HER, AND SO SHE LEFT IN HARRY. WELL I SAYED TO MYSELF < MMM... JUST IN TIME, PRAISE THE LORD! >. AFTER THAT I THANKED THE NURSES

IN THE RECEPTION, WHERE THERE WAS AN ENGLISH PATIENT CURSING THEM AND ME; AND SO EXPLAINING TO THEM THAT I HAD FINISHED MY WORK, I LEFT THE WARD AND HOSPITAL TO GO TO HAVE A SNACK AND SOME TEA, AND FIND OTHER PEOPLE TO WITNESS TO BEFORE EVENING SERVICE.

HOWEVER THE LORD DOES NOT FORGET US WHEN WE VISIT THE SICK, THE PRISONERS AND THE MARGINALISED [MATTH 25:31-46]. NOR WE MUST BE ARROGANT WHEN WE SERVE HIM BECAUASE IT IS ONLY BY HIS GRACE THAT WE DO IT; SO IN WHATEVER WE DO WE ARE GREATFUL IN THE PRIVILEDGE OF PARTAKING IN HIS WORK, AS WELL AS WE ENJOY HIS BLESSING NOW AND IN ETERNITY. I MUST SAY I WAS ALSO QUITE IMPRESSED AS FROM SUNDAY TO TUESDAY I HAD MY HEAD STICKY AS IT HAD BEEN ANOINTED WITH OIL, AND CERTAINLY WAS NOT SWEAT SINCE THE WEATHER WAS COOL AND RATHER A BIT CHILLY TOO. IN FACT I REMEMBER TO BE ON DUTY ON MONDAY; BUT EVEN ON TUESDAY EVENING, BEING OFF WORK, I THINK I MUST HAVE BEEN SHINING TOO AS SOME PEOPLE DURING THESE BOTH DAYS, HAD BEEN STARING AT ME WITH A LITTLE WONDER AND PLEASURE!

OBVIOUSLY WE SHOULD NOT BE TOO SURPRISED AT THIS AS WE ARE THE SALT AND LIGHT OF THE EARTH, AND WE ARE BEING TRANSFORMED INTO HIS IMAGE FROM GLORY TO GLORY AND ARE GETTING CLOSER TO RECIEVING FROM THE LORD THE CROWN OF LIFE AS IN MATTH 5:13-16 AND IN REV 2:8-11; AND FINALLY IN 2 COR 3:18 READS: < BUT WE ALL, WITH UNVEILED FACE, BEHOLDING AS IN A

MIRROW THE GLORY OF THE LORD, ARE BEING TRANSFORMED INTO THE SAME IMAGE FROM GLORY TO GLORY, JUST AS BY THE SPIRIT OF THE LORD > .

THUS, TO HIM BE GLORY, POWER AND HONOR FOR EVER AND EVER, AMEN!

****

AS I FINISH THIS CHAPTHER I WOULD LIKE TO BLESS YOU WITH A LAST LITTLE STORY. THE FOLLOWING EVENT HAPPENED PERHAPS AT THE END OF 2013. DURING THE DAY I HAD DONE A LOT OF OUTREACH WORK IN THE STREETS SHARING THE GOSPEL WITH AL KIND OF PEOPLE AND NATIONALITIES, AND ALL THIS IN PEACEFUL CONVERSATIONS AND DEBATES. IN THE EVENINING I HAD MANAGED TO HAVE SOME READING, PEACEFUL AND RELAXED TIME, PERHAPS MEETING MORE PEOPLE AND CHATTING IN A MORE RELAXED WAY. I REMEMBER TO HAVE GONE HOME AT ABOUT MIDNIGHT.

NOW AS I ENTERED THE HOUSE, I DIRECTED MYSELF TOWARDS MY BEDROOM; SUDDENLY AS I OPENED THE DOOR AND WENT IN, I HEARD A VOICE AS SAYING TO ME "A MONSTER, THERE IS A MONSTER HERE"!

AS I HEARD THE VOICE, I KIND OF STOOD STILL AND GATHERED MYSELF, THEN I BEGAN TO LOOK AROUND IN

THIS MEDIUM SIZE BEDROOM AND I COULD NOT SEE ANYTHING/ONE UNUSUAL.

I MUST SAY THAT I WAS NOT TOO WORRIED DESPITE THE VOICE, HAVING EXPERIENCED THE GRACE OF GOD IN MANY WAYS, AND SOMEHOW I HAD FELT THAT IT WAS THE VOICE OF THE HOLY SPIRIT.

AND SO I WENT TO BED TO REST AND STARTED TO READ THE BIBLE OR SOME CHRISTIAN BOOKS. HOWEVER I WAS STILL THINKING ABOUT THIS VOICE, AND IF REALLY THERE WAS AN UNWANTED GUEST IN MY BEDROOM. I GUESSED I WAS NOT TOO WORRIED BECAUSE IT WAS NOT JUST THE TWO OF US THERE, BUT REALLY THREE: ME, THE MONSTER, AND THE LORD!

SUDDENLY AS I WAS READING, SOMETHING MADE ME LOOK UP, AND THERE IT WAS: A HUGE SPIDER, THE BIGGEST I HAD EVER SEEN, AND TO BE MORE PRECISE, I THINK IT WA THE SAME ONE THAT I HAD SEEN A FEW DAYS BEFORE FOR A FRACTION OF A SECOND HIDING BEHIND THE TOILET SEAT, THE ONLY THING THIS TIME IT WAS IN MY BEDROOM. NOW I REMEMBER TALKING SOME MONTHS AFTER WITH AN ENGLISH WOMAN ABOUT IT AND SHE TOLD ME THAT THESE SPIDERS ARE OFTEN CALLED "WHOPPERS"; SHE FURTHER EXPLAINED TO ME THAT THEY COME FROM AFRICA IN THE CASKS OF BANANAS [MAYBE THE EGGS TOO]. I HEARD BY SOME THAT ARE POISONOUS TOO.

ANYHOW THERE IT WAS RUNNING AWAY FROM ME ON THE CARPET NEXT TO MY BED. HIS BODY ONLY MUST HAVE BEEN AT LEAST 2CM. + THICK LONG LEGS TOO. THEN I QUICKLY REALISED THAT IT MUST HAVE BEEN THE "MONSTER"; WITH NO CHOICE AND SOME COURAGE I HAD TO GET UP IN A HURRY AND REMOVE IT FROM MY ROOM SO THAT I COULD REST WELL!

WELL FUNNY ENOUGH SOME MONTHS LATER I REMEMBER SHARING THIS STORY WITH A SPANISH WOMAN. I RECALL TELLING HER THE PARTICULAR THAT I STILL HAD DECIDED TO GO TO BED TO REST DESPITE THIS SUSPICIOUS PRESENCE, AND HAVING STOPPED ME SHE EXCLAIMED " YOU WENT TO BED..., IF I HAD KNOWN THE WAS A MONSTER IN MY BEDROOM, I WOULD HAVE GOT MY PASSPORT AND LEFT THE HOUSE! WELL...WHAT CAN WE SAY...?

BASICALLY I THEN UNDERSTOOD THAT IT HAD BEEN THE HOLY SPIRIT WARNING ME THAT THERE WAS AN ENEMY/MONSTER IN MY ROOM; AND SO I REMEMBER THAT HE GUIDES US TO THE TRUTH, AND TAKES WHAT BELONG TO THE LORD JESUS AND REVEALS IT TO US AS THE GOSPEL OF JOHN 16:13-14 TELLS US SO, TO THE GLORY OF GOD AMEN!

==

4   SINISTER ACTIVITIES

PART A

I CERTAINLY DO NOT FIND EXCITING TO SPEAK ABOUT DEMONIC ACTIVITIES AND ENCOUNTERS, FOR UNFORTUNATELY IT IS MAINLY BECAUSE OF THE REAL PRESENCE OF THESE, AND THE HUMAN TENDENCY TO BE UNAWARE OF THEIR OPERATIONS, AND SO INDEED TO PLAY THEIR GAMES AND SUCCUMB TO THEM, THAT THE HUMAN CONDITIONS ON EARTH ARE RATHER DRAMATIC AND PITIFUL; ACTUALLY THESE CONDITIONS ARE ULTIMATELY FATAL ENDING IN DEATH FOR ALL HUMAN BEINGS, VERELY SO FOR THE DEVIL HAVING THE POWER OF DEATH AS WE CAN SEE IN HEBR 2:14-15: < INASMUCH AS THE CHILDREN HAVE PARTAKEN OF FLESH AND BLOOD, HE HIMSELF LIKEWISE SHARED IN THE SAME, THAT THROUGH DEATH HE MIGHT DESTROY HIM WHO HAD THE POWER OF DEATH, THAT IS, THE DEVIL...>

THUS WE REJOICE AND ARE THANKFUL FOR THE RESURRECTION OF JESUS!!!

HAVING MADE THIS BOTH SIMPLE AND PROFOUND COMMENT, I WOULD LIKE TO BIGIN THIS FOURTH CHAPTER WITH A SIMPLE BUT I BELIEVE ALSO VERY IMPORTANT AND RELEVANT STORY FOR US TODAY. THIS EPISODE MUST HAVE OCCURRED PERHAPS ABOUT FIFTEEN YEARS AGO', AND WITHOUT DOUBT I MUST HAVE BEEN ATTENDING BIBLE COLLEGE. FOR YEARS I HAVE BEEN GOING TO THE SAME SHOES REPAIRER, NOT FAR FROM THE AREAS WHERE I USUALLY LIVE, AND I HAVE ALWAYS MANTAINED A GOOD RELATIONSHIP WITH

THE MAN WHO IS FROM ASIA, WHO I MUST SAY IS ALWAYS VERY KIND TO ME TOO. HAVING BECOME A COMMITTED BELIEVER, I ALSO STARTED TO WITNESS TO HIM AND INVITE HIM TO OUR CHURCH EVERY NOW AND AGAIN. I THINK THAT, THOUGH IN A POLITE MANNER HE NEVER REALLY PAYED MUCH ATTENTION TO ME, AND HE DID NOT SEEM TO BE VERY INTERESTED IN HIS OWN RELIGION TOO; I THINK OF HIM, RATHER THAN A MUSLIM FROM PAKISTAN, MORE LIKE A SECULAR LONDONER. I REMEMBER THAT SOMETIMES HE ALSO USED TO THANK ME, MAY BE ESPECIALLY BECAUSE I USED TO INFORM HIM THAT IN OUR CHURCH WE WERE SEEING MANY HEALINGS, THUS IF HE HAD ANY RELATIVES OR FRIENDS IN PAIN OR WITH SICKNESS, PLEASE TO LET THEM KNOW ABOUT IT.

WELL IT IS CERTAINLY A BIG CHALLENGE WHEN WE START TO THINK ABOUT ALL THE ENORMOUS WORK THAT NEEDS TO BE DONE ON THIS PLANET.

NOW WHAT WAS INTERESTING ABOUT ALL THIS IS THAT ONE DAY HAPPENED SOMETHING DIFFERENT AND UNUSUAL. I WAS IN FACT GOING TO SEE HIM AS I HAD SOME SHOES TO REPAIR. AS I WAS HEADING TOWARDS HIS SHOP, MAYBE A 3-4 METERS AWAY, I COULD SEE HIM ALREADY THERE WORKING AS USUAL. THIS TIME HOWEVER, AS I WAS GETTING CLOSER, VERY STRANGELY HE WAS STARING AT ME LOOKING VERY UPSET OR DISTURBED AGAINST ME! QUITE SURPRISED I BEGAN TO WONDER WHAT IT WAS ALL ABOUT. ANYHOW IN CONFIDENCE I WENT IN SHOWING A NICE FACE, AND THE

LOOK OF HIS FACE BECAME FRIENDLY AND WE GENTLY GREETED EACH OTHER AS USUALLY. HOWEVER, AS IT HAPPENED I WAS UNDER THE POWER OF THE HOLY SPIRIT, I BELIEVE UNDER HIS GIFT OF DISCERNMENT [I COR 12]; IN FACT AS I LOOK AROUND INSIDE HIS SHOP SOMETHING IMPORTANT WAS HAPPENING. AS I WAS FACING THE MAN, ON MY RIGHT HAND SIDE AT ABOUT TWO METERS AND HALF IN HEIGHT, I SAW LIKE TWO VERY BRIGHT, LIKE YELLOWISH SPOTS HANGING/APPEARING IN THE AIR. EACH PERHAPS WAS ABOUT I-2 CENTEMETER IN DIAMETER. UNFORTUNATELY I CAN NOT REMEMBER PRECISELY NOW WHAT WAS THE DISTANCE BETWEEN THEM, BUT I DO NOT THINK MORE THAN A METER, AND MORE LIKELY CLOSER THAN THAT. THIS WAS NOT ALL; IN THE ROOM, AS I WAS JUST INSIDE THE SHOP, THERE WAS A LOUD VOICE SHOUTING < HIM, HIM, HIM...>. THIS LASTED JUST FOR A FEW SECONDS.

BASICALLY THIS VOICE WAS ACCUSING ME BEFORE THE MAN WITH THE PURPOSE OF INCITING THAT DEAR MAN TO GO AGAINST ME, AND SO STOP OUR RELATIONSHIP AND THE VARIOUS OPPORTUNITIES TO SAVE HIS LIFE WITH THE GOSPEL. THUS THIS VOICE WAS OF THAT DEMON THERE, WHO WAS STANDING OR IN THE AIR, AT MY RIGHT HAND, WHERE THE TWO SPOTS WERE [SEE ZECH. 3:1-3; AND REV 12:10].

THOUGH I CAN NOT EXPLAIN THE TWO SPOTS IN THE AIR, AS I AM NOT SURE IN TRUTH, MAYBE THEY WERE THE EYES OF THAT EVIL SPIRIT, AND IF THAT IS THE CASE HIS STATURE COULD HAVE BEEN AT ALMOST 3 METERS;

BUT I AM SPECULATING HERE, AS THESE ARE SPIRITS AND THEY MAY NOT HAVE EYES AT ALL!?!

THOUGH NOT TALKING ABOUT ANGELS, WE KNOW ABOUT GIANTS IN THE SCRIPTURES [GEN. 6]. BY THE WAY IN THIS LAST BIBLICAL REFERENCE, WE MUST OBSERVE A LINK WITH SEXUAL IMMORALITY, WHICH I WANT TO STRESS AGAIN THAT IT IS STILL A TERRIBLE PROBLEM OF SOCIETY TODAY.

ANYHOW I HAD SOON REALISED THAT IT WAS FOR THIS SPIRITUAL SITUATION THAT THE MAN AT FIRST WAS LOOKING DISTURBED AND ANGRY AT ME. OBVIOUSLY THE POOR MAN HAD NOT SEEN NOR HEARD ANYTHING OF WHAT I WAS ENABLED TO DISCERN [BY THE HOLY SPIRIT], SEE, AND HEAR CLEARLY ABOUT WHAT WAS HAPPENING SPIRITUALLY IN HIS SHOP!

I KEPT IN CONTROL HAVING SOUND BIBLICAL KNOWLEDGE AND HAVING THE HOLY SPIRIT WITH AND IN ME. AFTERWARDS WE CONTINUE TO SPEAK ABOUT MY SHOES TO BE REPAIRED AND THE USUAL THINGS AS NOTHING HAD HAPPENED.

AS BELIEVERS WE MUST BE AWARE THAT THE DEVIL IS THE ACCUSER AND ALWAYS TRYING TO CAUSE SEPARATIONS AND WORSEN RELATIONSHIPS BETWEEN PEOPLE.

IT IS GOOD TO REMEMBER HIS STRATEGIES AND PROMOTE RECONCILIATIONS. BUT HE ALSO ATTACKS US AT A PERSONAL LEVEL TO PUT US DOWN AND RENDER US INEFFICIENT IN OUR MINISTRY AND LIFE. HE LIES SO BY REMINDING US OF OUR PAST MISTAKES, WITH THE PURPOSE TO MAKE US FEEL GUILTY AND USELESS. HOWEVER AS SOME WOULD SAY, WHEN THE DEVIL DOES THIS, WE SHOULD ALSO REMIND HIM OF HIS FUTURE DESTINATION, AS WELL AS REMINDING OURSELVES THAT THE BLOOD OF THE LAMB HAS WASHED US TOTALLY, AND PURGED OUR CONSCIENCE ENABLING US TO CONTINUALLY SERVE THE LIVING GOD AS HEBR 9:11-15 TELLS US: <...HOW MUCH MORE SHALL THE BLOOD OF CHRIST, WHO THROUGH THE ETERNAL SPIRIT OFFERED HIMSELF WITHOUT SPOT TO GOD, CLEANSE YOUR CONSCIENCE FROM DEAD WORKS TO SERVE THE LIVING GOD?...>

I MUST ALSO CONFESS TO YOU THAT DESPITE MY STANDING IN CHRIST, I WAS ONLY ABLE TO GO AND SHARE THIS SPIRITUAL DIMENSION AND EVENT WITH THE SAME MAN AT LEAST AFTER ABOUT TWO YEARS; I WAS IN FACT SCARED TO DO THIS BEFORE, SUCH IT HAD IMPACTED ME. THE EVENT INDEED HAD A VIOLENT NATURE: THAT DEMON WAS VERBALLY VIOLENT! BUT NO MATTER WHAT, I DID GO BACK THERE.

MOREOVER OBEYING GOD AND HIS SCRIPTURES BRING TO US MORE BLESSINGS TOO.

FINALLY AND SADLY, EVEN AFTER TELLING THIS STORY TO THE MAN, THIS SHOWED NO MUCH INTEREST IN ANYTHING. I DO NOT KNOW, BUT HIS HEART SEEMED HARD; FOR HIM IT IS OK FOR EVERYBODY TO FOLLOW HIS OWN PATH. STILL I HOPE HE WILL MAKE IT TO HEAVEN. IN RECALLING THIS STORY, I THINK WE NEED TO REMEMBER TO BE MORE SPIRITUALLY SENSITIVE AND AWAKE, SINCE WE ARE CALLED TO WALK BY FAITH AND NOT BY SIGHT [2 COR 4:16-18; 5:7].

****

THE NEXT EPISODE I AM ABOUT TO WRITE TO YOU ABOUT, I BELIEVE IS WORTHY OF CAREFUL ANALYSIS AND THOUGHT, AS OFTEN WE DO NOT KNOW WHERE IN OUR DAILY LIFE WE RELLY PUT OUR HANDS ON,
NOT FORSEEING THE FOLLOWING COSEQUENCES OF OUR ACTIONS !

I THINK FOR ABOUT 7-8 YEARS I HAVE BEEN KNOWN A JEWISH LADY WHO, AS A SIDE JOB WOULD READ CARDS AND TELL THE FUTURE TO VARIOUS CLIENTS BOTH REGULAR AND NEW. I TOOK IT UPON ME TO TALK TO HER, KNOWING FROM THE SCRIPTURES THAT THESE ARE NOT GOOD PRACTISES TO INDULGE IN [DEUT. 18].

AND SO I BEGAN TO CHAT HER UP, BEING ALSO A GOOD LOOKING WOMAN TOO [SORRY BUT TRUE]. EVERY NOW

AND THEN I WOULD WITNESS TO HER, AND AT TIMES
EVEN HELPED HER WITH HER BAGS. AFTER ABOUT TWO
YEARS I ONCE TOOK HER TO MY CHURCH SINCE SHE HAD
INFORMED ME OF SOME KIND OF HEARING CONDITION
THAT WAS BOTHERING HER FOR SOMETIMES. I RECALL IT
MUST HAVE BEEN ON A SATURDAY AND SHE HAD
ENJOYED THE SERVICE, THOUGH SHE REMAINED STILL
RESISTANT TO THE GOSPEL. SHE ALSO TOLD ME
SOMETHING INTERESTING: IN THE NIGHT SHE WAS
SUFFERING FROM THE BAD HABIT OF BITING HER
TOUNGUE WITH HER TEETH, AND THEREFORE SHE
WOULD HAVE TO SLEEP WEARING IN HER MOUTH AN
OBJECT OF PLASTIC/RUBBER FOR PROTECTION. THIS
STRAIGHTAWAY REMINDED ME OF JESUS' WARNING OF
THE FUTURE GNASHING OF TEETH, AS ONE OF THE
CONDITIONS OF PEOPLE IN ETERNAL CONDEMNATION AS
IN MATTH 8:12: < "BUT THE SONS OF THE KINGDOM WILL
BE CAST IN OUTER DARKNESS. THERE WILL BE WEEPING
AND GNASHING OF TEETH." >

WELL YOU WILL BE PLEASED TO KNOW, THAT
BEING BIBLICALLY FAIRLY EQUIPPED, I ALWAYS KEPT A
CERTAIN RESPECTFUL DISTANCE FROM HER, AND NEVER
CAME THE OCCASION TO VISIT HER FRIEND AND HER
HOUSE.

NOW IT MUST HAVE BEEN ABOUT 3-4 YEARS AGO' THAT
SOMETHING VERY INTERESTING HAPPENED. I WAS STILL
CO-PASTORING THE SATELLITE CHURCH WITH MEMBERS
MOSTLY FROM SIERRA LEONE; I WAS ALSO ATTENDING
THE MAIN CHURCH. AS I HAVE ALREDY MENTIONED

ABOVE, SHE WAS AND STILL IS AN ATTRACTIVE WOMAN, SAVED WHEN SHE GET DRESSED A BIT TOO LOOSE SHOWING 3/5 OF HER BREASTS, THEN IN MY OPINION, SHE LOOSES MUCH OF HER ELEGANCE, AS SHE SO SHOWS TOO LITTLE OF HERSELF! AS YOU ALSO KONW PAUL WARNS US TO TAKE HEED WHEN WE THINK WE STAND LEST WE FALL [1 COR. 10:12].

ANYHOW MOVING ON, THIS TIME I WAS IN MY HOME; I WAS IN BED RESTING AT NIGHT TRYING TO GET SOME SLEEP. I WAS STILL CLEARLY AWAKE AND SOME DISTURBING TOUGHTS WERE PASSING THROUGH MY MIND. IN TRUE HONESTY, NOT BEING GLORIFIED JET, I WAS ALSO THINKING ABOUT THIS LADY, THE FORTUNE TELLER, KNOWING ALSO THAT SHE LIKED ME TOO. I AM AFRAID SOME THOUGHTS WERE NOT GODLY AT ALL, AS SOMETIMES AT NIGHT WE CAN FEEL A LITTLE WEAK. IN THOSE MOMENTS I WAS GETTING ENTICED, IN MY MIND AS I WAS BIGINNING TO BE DRAWN AWAY; JUST THINK THERE I HAD STARTED TO DOUBT EVEN WHETHER THESE FORTUNE TELLING AND SO ON PRACTICES, WERE WRONG AND CARRIED SERIOUS CONSEQUENCES OR NOT. SUDDENLY AS THESE THOUGHTS WERE CROSSING SLOWLY MY MIND, AN EVIL SPIRIT CAME INSIDE MY BED. I REMEMBER LYING IN MY BED ON MY LEFT SIDE, AND TO MY SHOCK AND RATHER DISPLEASURE, I CLEARLY FELT THE SPIRIT LYING JUST BEHIND ME ON HIS LEFT SIDE AND VERY CLOSE TO ME!

LIKE A MARRIED COUPLE IN LOVE I ALSO FELT HIM PUTTING HIS SPIRITUAL ARMS AROUND MY SHOULDERS

CADDLING ME. AS YOU CAN UNDERSTAND, WE CHRISTIAN CAN BE VERY FUSSY IN CHOOSING OUR WIVES!!!

HAVING HAD EXPERIENCES WITH DEMONS BEFORE, AND KONWING MY STANDING IN CHRIST, I DID NOT PANIC AND I KEPT IN CONTROL, BUT I FELT AS I WAS ALLERGIC TO THIS NOCTURNAL COMPANY. I MUST CONFESS TO YOU THAT THERE WAS NO ROMANCE BETWEEN US HOWEVER, NOT FROM HIS PART EITHER. HE SPOKE NO WORDS TO ME, BUT HE STARTED TO LAUGH AT ME FROM BEHIND, WITH SOUNDS THAT WERE SCOFFING AND MOCKING ME [PLEASE SEE PSALM 1]. I DID NOT SAY ANYTHING TO HIM, AND I BEGAN TO PULL MYSELF TOGETHER IN UNDERSTANDING AND REASONING, KNOWING THAT THIS SPIRIT HAD COME BECAUSE OF MY SINFUL AND DOUBTFUL THOUGHTS. THEN WITH THE AUTHORITY THAT WE HAVE IN CHRIST I REBUKED HIM AND COMMANDED HIM TO GET OUT OF MY BED AND TO LEAVE MY ROOM. TO MY CONFORT AND PEACE, STRAIGHT AWAY THE EVIL SPIRIT LEFT BOTH MY BED AND MY ROOM. THOUGH IT WAS NOT BRIGHT IN THE ROOM, I HAD THE STRONG SENSATION THAT HE LEFT THE ROOM FROM MY LEFT HANDSIDE THROUGH THE EXTERNAL WALL LEADING OUTSIDE WHICH WAS NEAR MY BED.

WELL THIS EXPERIENCE WAS CERTAINLY REASSURING FOR ME THAT I WAS TO BE VERY CAREFUL IN HOW TO EVANGELISE THIS LADY; NOT THAT I HAD REALLY DOUBTED THE WORD OF GOD, BUT WE ALWAYS NEED LESSONS FROM GOD AS WE DO HIS WORK AND WALK IN

THIS VERY MUCH DEMONISED WORLD, AS WE CAN CLEARLY OBSERVE IN 2 COR 10 AND EPH 6:11-12 WHICH READS: < PUT ON THE ALL ARMOUR OF GOD, THAT YOU MAY BE ABLE TO STAND AGAINST THE WILES OF THE DEVIL. FOR WE DO NOT WRESTLE AGAINST FLESH AND BLOOD, BUT AGAINST PRICIPALITIES, AGAINST POWERS, AGAINST THE RULERS OF THE DARKNESS OF THIS AGE, AGAINST SPIRITUAL HOSTS OF WICKEDNESS IN THE HEAVENLY PLACES. >

I SINCERELY HOPE THAT TELLING YOU OF THIS OTHER EXPERIENCE OF MINE HAS BEEN A BLESSING TO YOU AND HAS GIVING YOU SOME GOOD FOOD FOR THOUGHT, AND WE NEED ALL THE FOOD THAT WE CAN DIGEST SO THAT WE CAN STAND FIRM EVEN IN THIS DIFFICULT AGE!

BY THE WAY I HAVE NOT SEEN THIS PERSON FOR SOME TIME, AS SHE MAY BE WORKING IN A DIFFERENT PLACE. I PRAY THAT ONE DAY GOD WILL OPEN HER EYES AND ENABLE HER TO SEE HIS SALVATION, TO THE GLORY OF THE FATHER, IN JESUS' WONDERFUL NAME, AMEN!

****

AT THIS POINT I WOULD LIKE TO TELL YOU OF AN OTHER EVENT, I BELIEVE ALSO QUITE INTERESTING AND

INSPIRATIONAL SOMEHOW, THAT HAPPENED TO ME POSSIBLY AROUND FIFTEEN YEARS AGO'. THIS STORY REALLY TAKES PLACE BOTH HERE IN LONDON AS WELL AS IN ITALY IN MY SMALL TOWN. QUITE LIKELY I WAS STILL IN BIBLE COLLEGE, DOING A LOT OF WITNESSING, AND A GOOD AMOUNT OF PRAYER TOO; I REMEMBER BEING QUITE STRONG AND ZELOUS IN SPIRIT AND UNDER HIS ANOINTING. WELL ANYHOW IT HAPPENED THAT DURING AN EVENING FREE FROM WORK, THAT I WAS STANDING OUTSIDE A LARGE AND REKNOWN STORE IN CENTRAL LONDON NEAR OXFORD STREET; THERE I BEGAN TO TALK WITH A MAN FROM NIGERIA WHO WAS STANDING NEXT TO HIS RATHER LARGE AND EXPENSIVE CAR. NOW THIS MAN MUST HAVE BEEN WAITING FOR HIS WIFE WHO CAME AFTER, AND FUNNY ENOUGH I HAD ALREADY MET AND WITNESSED TO HER IN THE PAST.

NOW I WAS HAVING A GOOD CHAT WITH THIS MAN ABOUT GOD, RELIGION AND MY CHURCH, BUT I THINK IT WAS AFTER HIS WIFE CAME AND LEFT THAT WE BEGAN TO BE A LITTLE MORE PERSONAL. BASICALLY HE STARTED TO TELL ME THAT HE HAD A WEAK AND BAD HABIT: WOMEN! AND THAT HE COULD NOT HELP HIMSELF, THOUGH HE FELT GUILTY AT TIMES. WELL TO CUT THE STORY SHORT, I WAS NOT PLEASED WITH THAT, AND I BEGAN TO BOTH ENCOURAGE HIM AND TELL HIM OFF AT THE SAME TIME. I THINK I DID SO, PEHAPS IN A WAY LIKE THE APOSTLE PAUL IN HIS LETTERS DID, WHEN HE USED TO PRAY/PRAISE THE NEW BELIEVERS AND THEN REBUKE THEM AND LECTURE THEM [EX. 1 COR 1; 5].

I BRIEFLY WANT TO PAUSE HERE AS I DESIRE AGAIN TO
REMEMBER AGAIN THIS PROBLEM OF IMMORALITY
TODAY AS IN ALL HUMAN HISTORY,
SOMETHING EVIDENCED THROUGHOUT THE SCRIPTURES.

AND SO IN MANY WAYS I TRIED TO ENCOURAGE HIM IN
THE CHRISTIAN FAITH, IN LIVING A HOLY MARRIAGE AND
VISIT OUR CHURCH, AND IF LIKED IT, GET INVOLVED IN ITS
MINISTRY TOO. HE TOLD ME THAT HE CAME FROM AN
INPORTANT FAMILY IN HIS COUNTRY AND WAS LIVING IN
A NICE AREA HERE IN LONDON, AND HE ALSO INVITED ME
TO TAKE ME TO HIS HOUSE WHEN I WANTED TO. NOW I
DID NOT FEEL LED TO PURSUE THIS RELATIONSHIP, BUT I
DID HOPE THAT OUR MEETING CONVICTED HIM AND
BLESSED HIM SOMEHOW, AND HELPED HIM TO BE
ROOTED IN ANY GOOD CHURCH.

NOW WHEN THE TIME CAME FOR MY NEXT HOLIDAYS, AS
USUALLY I WOULD BE GOING TO VISIT MY FAMILY IN
ITALY. SO THERE I WAS IN MY VILLAGE TO VISIT MY
FAMILY. AT THE TABLE HAVING DINNER OR LUNCH I
RECALLED THIS STORY TO MY FAMILY AS WELL AS
TALKING ABOUT DIFFERENT FAMILY AFFAIRS AND OTHER
TOPICS. MY FATHER WAS STILL ALIVE THEN, AND HE ALSO
LIKED TO TELL AND TO LISTEN TO STORIES; BY THE WAY
HE DIED AT THE AGE OF 89 IN 2000; TODAY HE WOULD
HAVE BEEN 100 YEARS OLD FROM FEBRUARY. HAVING

FINISHED OUR MEAL AND THE GATHERING IN THE SITTING ROOM, I LEFT TO GO TO MY AND MY BROTHER BEDROOM. SUDDENLY AS I WAS STANDING OR WALKING IN THE MIDDLE OF THE ROOM, NEXT TO MY RIGHT EAR, A VOICE SPOKE TO ME VERY CLEARLY! THIS UNCLEAN SPIRIT [DEMON] TALKED TO ME IN THE DIALECT OF MY VILLAGE. I WILL TRANSLATE HIS UTTERANCE HERE IN A LESS RUDE WAY. WHAT HE HAD SAIED WAS << HEEH, YOU HAVE A STRONG SEXUAL ORGAN >>. NOW I DO NOT KNOW WHY HE HAD SAIED THAT TO ME AS I WAS LIVING A HOLY LIFE!

COULD HAVE BEEN BECAUSE I WAS BOASTING IN MY PREACHING TELLING THE STORY TO MY FAMILY IN THE SITTING ROOM BEFORE? I DO NOT THINK SO. IT IS TRUE THAT WE SHOULD NO BE ARROGANT BUT IN CHRIST WE CAN BOAST [1 COR 1:13]! I BELIEVE IT HAPPENED AS GOD ALLOWED ME IN THE SPIRIT TO HEAR THIS DEMONIC UTTERANCE, PEHAPS TO MAKE ME UNDERSTAND MORE SATAN'S SCHEME, EVEN POSSIBLY AS A REWARD FOR DOING HIS WORK, AND WITNESS IT TOO [EPH 6:11].

IN FACT JESUS PROMISES US WHO HAVE, THAT HE WILL GIVE US MORE, THAT IS ALSO KNOWLEGE AND UNDERSTANDING [MATTH 13:12]; AND AS HIS CHURCH, WE CAN BE CONFIDENT TO STAND SAFE ONLY IN HIM AND HIS WORDS.

CERTAINLY LIVING IN A CITY LIKE LONDON, AS IN CORINTH IN THE TIMES OF THE APOSTLE PAUL, WE NEED TO FACE THE REALITY OF THE TERRIBLE SEXUAL

IMMORALITY THAT IS GOING ON WITH ALL ITS DEVASTATING CONSEQUENCES.

THIS IS NOT THE TIME TO GO INTO THIS TOPIC AT DEAPTH, BUT BOTH IN THIS CITY AND IN MY VILLAGE AS WELL ALL OVER THE WORLD, MANY PEOPLE DO NOT KNOW BUT ARE PLAYING THE DEVIL'S GAME: THAT IS THEY ARE WRONGLY INDULGING IN SEXUAL IMMORALITY FOR MANY REASONS, AND OFTEN, LIKE THE DEVIL WANTED ME TO BOAST, THEY BOAST AND SHOW OFF BETWEEN THEIR FRIENDS ABOUT THEIR ACTIONS.

THE SCRIPTURES CLEARLY CONDEMNS SEXUAL IMMORALITY AS IT IS CONSIDERED SPIRITUAL AND PHYSICAL ADULTERY AND IDOLATRY, INVOLVING HUMAN SEMEN/BLOOD [1COR 6:12-20]. THOUGH I RESPECT PEOPLE' FREEDOM OF OPINIONS AND ACTIONS, I BELIEVE ALSO THAT IT IS VERY WRONG AND DAMAGING; AND THAT THESE SHOW LACK OF WISDOM AS WELL AS LACK OF SPIRITUAL INSIGHT. TO PUT IT IN BIBLICAL TERMS, EVIL SPIRITS CAUSE A SPIRITUAL BLINDNESS AS PAUL INFORMS US IN 2 COR 4:3-4: < BUT EVEN IF OUR GOSPEL IS VEILED, IT IS VEILED TO THOSE WHO ARE PERISHING, WHOSE MINDS THE GOD OF THIS AGE HAS BLINDED, WHO DO NOT BELIEVE, LEST THE LIGHT OF THE GOSPEL OF THE GLORY OF CHRIST, WHO IS THE IMAGE OF GOD, SHOULD SHINE ON THEM. >

AGAIN OUR PRAYER IS THAT OUR LORD WOULD OPEN THE EYES OF THESE PEOPLE, THAT THEY WOULD REPENT

AND CALL ON THE NAME OF JESUS AND BE SAVED, TO
THE GLORY OF THE FATHER; AMEN [JOHN 3; ROM 10].

****

NEXT STORY I AM ABOUT TO TELL YOU NOW HAPPENED
TO ME PERHAPS AROUND 12/14 YEARS AGO'; THOUGH I
AM TRYING TO REMEMBER, I CAN NOT BE MORE PRECISE
THAN THIS, AND HOWEVER IT IS NOT TOO IMPORTANT IN
THIS OCCASION TO BE MORE PRECISE. IN FACT IT
MAY HAVE HAPPENED DURING MY YEARS OF BIBLE
COLLEGE FROM 95 TO 99, OR JUST AFTER.

ANY HOW IT IS SET IN THE RESTAURANT NEAR PICCADILLY
WHERE I WAS WORKING FOR SOME YEARS. AND SO
THERE WE WERE WORKING ONE EVENING AS USUALLY.

NOW, AS WE ALL KNOW IN OUR HUMAN IMPERFECTION,
IN OUR WORKING PLACES AT TIME WE CAN
HAVE VARIOUS ISSUES WITH BOTH OUR JOBS AND OUR
COLLEGUES, AFTER ALL WEL LIVE IN A FALLEN WORLD
DESPITE THE MANY SIGNS OF THE LORD'S WONDERFUL
GRACE IN IT. AND SO THE CASE WAS THAT I WAS FEELING
A LITTLE UPSET WITH A LADY COLLEGUE OF MINE, BUT
NOT REALLY HOLDING A GRUDGE OR BEING REALLY
BITTER AGAINST HER. THE REASON WAS THAT I THOUGHT
THAT SHE HAD BEING A BIT LAZY, I THINK THE EVENING
BEFORE, WHICH HAD CAUSED ME TO WORK HARDER,

AND PERHAPS TO FEEL MORE TIRED THE DAY AFTER, OBVIOUSLY. ANYHOW THAT EVENING WE STARTED TO WORK TOGETHER AS NORMALLY AND I WAS DOING MY BEST TO IGNORE THIS SMALL FEELING OF ANGER AGAINST HER, PUSHING IT ALMOST TO MY SUBCONSCIOUSNESS, IF I MAY SAY SO.

BUT AT A CERTAIN MOMENT OF THE EVENING SOMETHING INTERESTING HAPPENED, WHICH I THINK ALSO CAUSED ME TO DEAL WITH THIS TINY ALMOST HIDDEN SENSE OF UNFORGIVENESS TOWARDS HER.

NOW SHE WAS WORKING STANDING CLOSE TO ME AND SHE HAD TOLD ME THAT SHE WAS NOT FEELING WELL, BUT HAD A KIND OF COLD. WELL AT A CETAIN POINT, BELIEVE IT OR NOT, SHE SNEEZED! STRAIGHTAWAY AS YOU WOULD THINK, I SAYED TO HER << BLESS YOU >>. UNFORTUNATLY, WHAT HAD COME OUT OF ME WAS NOT REALLY A LOVING << BLESS YOU >>, BUT ALMOST RATHER THE OPPOSITE! THEN SUDDENLY TO MY WONDER, AS I HAD SAYED THAT TO HER, I FAIRLY CLEARLY SAW AROUND HER SOMETHING LIKE AN EVIL SPIRIT, WHO SUDDENLY REACTED TO MY WORDS, TURNED AND MADE A MOVE COMING CLOSER TOWARDS ME, LIKE IF HE WAS THREATENING TO JUMP ON ME TOO! NOW REGARDING MY COLLEGUE, SHE MUST HAVE SAYED THANK YOU TO ME AS NORMALLY, AND I BELIEVE SHE SAW NOTHING OF ALL THIS.

NOW I AM SURE THAT I NEED TO LEARN MORE ON THE
POWER OF WORDS, AND THE LORD JESUS SPEAK A LOT
ON WORDS IN THE GOSPELS.

FOR SURE I ASKED MYSELF WHAT DID THIS SCENERY
MEAN? AND I DID PONDER ON THE SIGNIFICANCE OF ALL
THIS. DO KNOW THAT AS I CONSIDERED IN THAT TIME,
STILL EVEN TODAY I THINK THAT THERE MAY HAVE BEEN
A LINK BETWEEN HER CONDITION OF HAVING A COLD OR
SOME KIND OF "FLU", AND THIS EVIL SPIRIT WHO WAS
SURROUNDING HER. INTERERSTINGLY I WAS ABLE TO
DISCERN THE DEMON ONLY AS HE MOVED
FAST TOWARDS ME ALMOST LIKE "A NEAR TO SHAPELESS
"MASS OF PERSONAL LIVING AIR, AS HE SHIFTED
SO AGGRESSIVELY TOWARDS ME. IT IS ALSO POSSIBLE
THAT AS I SPOKE << BLESS YOU >>; GOD'S PRESENCE
ENABLED ME TO DISCERN THIS, AS I WAS LIVING AN
ANOINTED LIFESTYLE.

NOW AS WE LOOK AT THE SCRIPTURES, WE OFTEN SEE
THE PRESENCE OF HUMAN CONDITIONS OF SICKNESSESS
LINKED WITH EVIL SPIRITS DIRECTLY; AT TIMES SOME
VERSES OF SCRIPTURES WOULD INCLUDE JESUS ACTIONS
OF EXORCISMS CLOSE TO REFERENCES OF HIM HEALING
DESEASES; OR EVEN AT TIMES REFERENCES OF JUST
HEALING DEASESES [MATTH 17:18; 8:16; 8:15; 9:1-8].
NOTE INTERESTINGLY IN THE LAST TWO REFERENCES,
FIRST THE ACTIVE WORDS < THE FEVER LEFT HER >,
AND IN THE LAST THE CLEAR CONNECTION OF THE

PARALYTIC CONDITION WITH SIN [AT LEAST HERE ANYHOW]; V.6 IN FACT READS AS FOLLOWS: < "BUT THAT YOU MAY KNOW THAT THE SON OF MAN HAS POWER ON EARTH TO FORGIVS SINS"- THEN HE SAID TO THE PARALYTIC, "ARISE, TAKE UP YOUR BED, AND GO TO YOUR HOUSE." > JUST WONDERFUL!

NOW REFLECTING FEW SECONDS AGAIN, SEEING JESUS IN HIS MINISTRY IS FASCINATING, AND IT CALLS US TO ACTION!

HAVING SAID THIS, I THINK THAT I NEED TO BE CAREFUL AND I CANNOT SAY THAT ALL SICKNESSES ARE DIRECTLY LINKED WITH DEMONIC ACTIVITIES, BECAUSE WE ALSO KNOW THAT THE GROUND WAS CURSED BECAUSE OF SIN CAUSING CHAOS AND CONFUSION IN THE UNIVERSE; AS WE SEE FOR EXAMPLE SO MANY EARTHQUAKES, EXTREME WEATHER CONDITIONS, ETC... BUT AT THE SAME TIME I WOULD LIKE TO REFLECT AND SAY THAT IT WAS CURSED BECAUSE OF OUR SINS CAUSED BY THE DEMONIC ACTIVITY IN THE ANCIENT GARDEN!!

MOREOVER I WOULD LIKE TO ADD THAT DEUTORONOMY MAKES IT CLEAR TO US THAT THINGS HAPPEN FOR A REASON ALWAYS, THAT THE LORD IS SOVEREIGN AND CAN PREVENT THEM, AND THAT HE IS OUR HEALER TO [DEUT. 28]! BUT LET US SEE TOGETHER JUST 2 VERSES OF THIS MAJESTIC BOOK, WHICH THE LORD JESUS ALSO USED TO BOTH DEFEND HIMSELF AND TO REBUKE THE DEVIL

WITH IN THE WILDERNESS [4:1-13]. HERE IS DEUT. 28:1;15 FOR US: < "NOW IT SHALL COME TO PASS, IF YOU DILIGENTLY OBEY THE VOICE OF THE LORD YOUR GOD...THE LORD YOUR GOD WILL SET YOU HIGH ABOVE ALL NATIONS OF THE EARTH......."BUT IT SHALL COME TO PASS, IF YOU DO NOT OBEY THE VOICE OF THE LORD YOUR GOD, TO OBSERVE CAREFULLY ALL HIS COMMANDMENTS AND HIS STATUTES WHICH I COMMAND YOU TODAY, THAT ALL THESE CURSES WILL COME UPON YOU AND OVERTAKE YOU: > SO HERE WE CAN REALLY SEE THAT THE LORD IS LORD, AND THAT HE MEANS REAL BUSINESS! WHETHER GOOD OR BAD BUSINESS WILL DEPEND MAINLY UPON US, AS WE OBEY HIM OR NOT!

I MAY BE WRONG BUT I STILL THINK THAT THIS COLLEGUE OF MINE HAD DONE SOMETHING BAD AND SO ATTRACTED THAT PARTICULAR DEMONIC CONDITION AND COLD ON HER!

NOT ONLY THIS, BUT AS I STILL THINK ABOUT IT, WHEN I SPOKE TO HER IN SUCH A NON-SINCERE WAY, ALMOST LIKE CURSING HER INSTEAD, THAT THIS DEMON FELT PROVOKED, AND TOOK MY WORDS AS A BRIDGE OR A PLATFORM TO TURN AT ME AND SO THREATENING TO ACT AGAINST ME TOO. IT WAS ALMOST LIKE IF HE WERE SAYING TO ME << DO YOU WANT PROBLEMS TOO? >>

I HOPE THIS STORY WILL BE OF INTEREST AND A BLESSING TO YOU. OF INPORTANCE IS THE FACT THAT FIRSTLY, NOW I AM MORE CAREFUL BOTH AT NOT HOLDING EVEN

SMALL GRUDGES AGAINST ANYONE, AND SECONDLY I
RECPECTFULLY REFLECT MORE WHEN SOMEBODY
SNEEZES BEFORE ME, BEFORE I SAY BLESS YOU TO THEM.

I MUST CONFESS TO YOU THAT I DO NOT THINK I EVER
TOLD HER THIS STORY, THOUGH I DID MENTION THIS TO
AN OTHER COLLEGUE OF MINE. I ALSO KEPT A GOOD
RELATIONSHIP WITH THIS LADY TILL SHE LEFT HER
POSITION. MAY GOD BLESS HER AS SHE WAS A FAIRLY
GOOD WOMAN.

****

WHAT I AM ABOUT TO TALK TO YOU NOW IS I BELIEVE A
POWERFUL SMALL STORY, ALMOST INCREDIBLE IF IT
WERE NOT JUSTIFIED BY THE SCRIPTURES; AND IT
HAPPENED ONLY ONCE TO ME. NOW THIS STORY MUST
HAVE TAKEN PLACE IN THE EARLY YEARS OF ME BEING IN
BIBLE COLLEGE, PERHAPS IN 95-96. IN THAT TIME I WAS
STAYING FOR SOME MONTHS WITH SOME CHURCH
FRIENDS IN THE AREA OF LADBROKE GROVE, HERE IN
LONDON. AS I SET THE SCENE, I MUST AGAIN SAY THAT IN
THOSE DAYS I WAS QUITE ZELOUS IN PRAYER,
INTERCESSION, SINGING, BIBLE READING, EVANGELIZING
AND TRYING TO TAKE TO CHURCH PEOPLE TOO. IT
HAPPENED THAT AT TIME, AS I STILL DO, I USED TO
SOCIALIZE WITH FRIENDS OF THE OPPOSITE SEX ALSO. I
OFTEN USED TO INTERCEDE FOR TWO LADIES IN

PARTICULAR, WHO WERE ALSO FRIENDS WITH THEMSELVES TOO: ONE WAS IRANIAN AND ONE WAS ITALIAN. THOUGH I MANAGED TO BRING BOTH OF THEM TO CHURCH WITH ME, NONE OF THEM WERE COMMITTED BELIEVERS; AS A MATTER OF FACT, UNFORTUNATELY, THEY WERE COMMITTED TO FINDING BOYFRIENDS FOR THEMSELVES. AT THAT TIME I WAS NOT AWARE, BUT THEY HAD BET £1,000 OVER MY HEAD, WITHOUT GOING INTO DETAILS. BEING MUCH YOUNGER AND MORE NAIVE THAN NOW, I WAS STILL SOCIALIZING A BIT TOO MUCH WITH THEM AT THE TIME, BUT IN THE FUTURE I STRAIGHTEN THINGS OUT, AVOIDING TO BE UNEQUALLY YOKED WITH THEM IN CLOSE RELATIONSHIPS. HOWEVER IN THE SPIRITUAL CONTEXT I WAS NOT PLEASED WITH THEIR BEHAVIOUR, AND EVEN LESS I WAS PLEASED WITH WHAT THE DEVIL WAS DOING TO THEM [SEE FOR EXAMPLE JOHN 4].

NOW IT IS POSSIBLE THAT I DO NOT REMEMBER FOR WHICH REASON I HAD GONE FOR A WALK OUTSIDE THE HOUSE, OR MOST LIKELY IT HAD HAPPENED THAT MORNING THAT I HAD GONE FOR A RUN AS I USUALLY STILL DO ONCE A WEEK. AFTER THE RUN I WOULD BE DOING SOME EXERCISES; AND SO THERE I WAS WALKING AROUND THE SMALL GREEN PIECE OF LAND NEAR THE HOUSE CALLED "WORMWOOD SCRUBS ". I STILL HAVE A VERY CLEAR MEMORY THAT AS I WAS WALKING I WAS INTERCEDING AND PRAYING REGARDING THIS ABOVE MENTIONED CONTEXT. AND, NOW BEING MORE

EXPERIENCED I DO NOT PRAY LIKE THIS ANYMORE, AS I WAS BEING RATHER HEAVVY ON THE DEVIL, SAYING THINGS LIKE << I AM GOING TO DESTROY YOU, ETC...>>, AND PERHAPS CALLING HIM NAMES.

BY THE WAY I STILL PRACTICE DELIVERANCE, AND CERTAINLY I AM NOT HIS FRIEND NOW [JUDE 9-10;]!!!

AND JOHN TELL US THAT JESUS CAME TO DESTROY THE WORK OF THE DEVIL [1 JOHN 3:8].

ANYHOW TO MY SHOCK, SUDDENLY I HEARD EXCATLY LIKE THE ROARING OF A LION NEAR MYSELF, AND I THINK THERE WAS NOBODY ELSE IN THE PARK AT THAT MOMEMENT, PERHAPS ONLY ONE OR TWO PEOPLE, RIGHT ON THE OTHER SIDE, AT ABOUT A HUNDRED YARDS AWAY!

SINCERELY, DESPITE KNOWING MY POSITION IN CHRIST AND THE HOLY SPIRIT IN ME, I MUST CONFESS TO YOU THAT IT WAS A SCARING EXPERIENCE; I HAD FELT SHAKEN, AND ALMOST STARTING TO MELT AND TO SWEAT. HIS IMPACT WAS WORSE AGAINST ME AS I DID NOT KNOW THAT SATAN IS LIKE A ROARING LION LOOKING FOR SOMEONE TO DEVOUR [1 PETER 5:8]. IN FACT I CAME ACROSS THIS SCRIPTURE IN MY BIBLE READING VARIOUS MONTHS AFTER EXPERIENCING THIS; HAD I READ THIS BEFORE I WOULD HAVE BEEN MORE PREPARED AND FELT NOT SO BAD.

NOTE THAT THE ROARING WAS SO REAL AS IF I HAD BEEN IN THE OPEN JUNGLE, OR IN A SAFARI, OR IN A ZOO, NEAR A WELL AWAKE AND ZELOUS LION WHILE HE WAS ROARING IN WRATH; OR EVEN MORE APPROPIATE MORE THAN JUST ZELOUS, BUT RATHER "JEALOUS" FOR HIS CHILDREN, OR FOR ANYBODY WHOM HE HAS IN HIS HANDS, NOT TO BE TAKEN AWAY FROM HIM! BUT SEE ON THE CONTRARY THE JELOUSY FOR US, OF THE REAL GOD OUR SAVIOUR IN JOHN 10:29; < "MY FATHER, WHO HAS GIVEN THEM TO ME, IS GREATER THAN ALL; AND NO NONE IS ABLE TO SNATCH THEM OUT OF MY FATHER'S HANDS. >

I THINK THAT IN THE LIGHT OF WHAT I JUST HAVE SAID, THIS BOTH WARNS AND ENCOURAGES US ALSO TO WALK IN HIS GRACE.

ANYWAY I DID NOT TAKE IT TOO BADLY, HAVING HAD ALREADY SOME OTHER SUPERNATURAL EXPERIENCES BEFORE AS A CHRISTIAN; AND SO I GUESS, AFTER FINISHING MY EXERCISES I MADE MY WAY BACK HOME. ALSO I GRADUALLY FOCUSED MORE IN GOD'S WORK AND SEPARATED MYSELF MORE FROM THESE TWO PARTICULAR PERSONS.

I AM HAPPY TO HAVE TOLD YOU THIS STORY, IN FACT AS I WRITE I AM ENCOURAGING MYSELF, AND I HOPE YOU TOO, TO CONTINUE TO PARTNER WITH GOD IN HIS MINISTRY OF MAKING DISCEPLES, OF BEING SALT AND LIGHT IN SOCIETY, AND IN DESTROYING THE WORK OF

THE DEVIL, KNOWING ALSO THAT HE DOES NOT HAVE A SOFT HAND ON HUMANITY AT ALL!

IN ADDITION I WOULD LIKE TO MAKE CLEAR THAT CERTAINLY FOR ME IN THE SCRIPTURES, ALL JESUS' STORIES, SUCH AS ALSO HIS DESCENT INTO HELL AND HIS ASCENSION, ARE PART OF HIS HISTORY AND LIFE; AND WITH RESPECT TOWARDS OTHER VIEWS, WE SHOULD TAKE THE SCRIPTURES IN A MORE REAL AND CONCRETE WAY, AS THEY USUALLY REALLY ARE!

THUS OUR AIM IS TO INFLUENCE OUR COMMUNITIES WITH THE VALUES OF THE KINGDOM OF GOD, BRINGING HIGHER LEVELS OF PEACE, SECURITY, AND WELL BEING HERE ON EARTH; THIS IN OPPOSITION TO THE SWAY OF THE WICKED ONE ON THIS GOD-CREATED AND OWNED EARTH, TO THE GLORY OF THE FATHER OF ALL MERCY AND GRACE AS WE CAN OBSERVE IN MATTH 5: 13-16; 28 AND 1 JOHN 3:8; 5:19-21, OF WHICH LAST THREE VERSES READ AS FOLLOWS: < AND WE KNOW THAT WE ARE OF GOD, AND THE ALL WORLD LIES UNDER THE SWAY OF THE WICKED ONE. AND WE KNOW THAT THE SON OF GOD HAS COME AND HAS GIVEN US AN UNDERSTANDING, THAT WE MAY KNOW HIM WHO IS TRUE; AND WE ARE IN HIM WHO IS TRUE, IN HIS SON JESUS CHRIST. THIS IS THE TRUE GOD AND ETERNAL LIFE. LITTLE CHILDREN, KEEP YOURSELVES FROM IDOLS. AMEN. >

=======================================
=

5 SINISTER ACTIVITIES

PART B

THE FOLLOWING STORY IS SET DURING THE PERIOD I WAS A PASTOR AT TOWER CHRISTIAN CENTRE, A SATELLITE CHURCH OF KENSINGTON TEMPLE HERE IN LONDON, FROM DEC- 2000 TO NOV-2007. NOW IN THIS PERIOD AMONG THE MANY ACTIVITIES I WAS INVOLVED IN THE CHURCH, SUCH AS PREACHING AND TEACHING, REGULARLY AND VERY MANY TIMES I WAS EVANGELISING IN THE SURROUNDING AREA. FOR REASON THAT I AM NOT AWARE, I MUST CONFESS TO YOU THAT MOST OF THE TIMES I USED TO END UP WITH BEING BY MYSELF IN THIS EVANGELISTIC ACTIVITY THERE, THOUGH I WOULD REGULARLY ADVERTISE IT IN THE CHURCH.

BUT I KNOW AND I AM SURE OTHER MEMBERS WERE QUITE ACTIVE IN DOING THIS IN OTHER AREAS AND WITH THEIR FRIENDS, AS THE CHURCH ATTENDANCE GREW FROM ABOUT 12 PEOPLE WHEN I STARTED TO ABOUT 45

AFTER NINE MONTHS BECAUSE OF GOD'S GRACE. I USED
TO DO THIS IN THE MAIN ROAD MOSTLY NEAR THE
BERMONDSEY UNDERGROUND STATION IN SOUTH
LONDON. I HAD NOTICED ALSO THAT THERE WERE SOME
ESTATES IN THE AREA WITH A FEW OF ITS DOORS
PROTECTED BY METAL BARS, MAKING ME REALIZE THAT
UNFORTUNATELY THE AREA SUFFERED SOME ISSUES
RELATED TO VIOLENCE, DRINKING AND PERHAPS RACISM.

ANYHOW I SPOKE TO MANY NICE PEOPLE IN THE AREA,
SOME OF WHOM WERE INTERESTED, AND WOULD EVEN
TAKE OUR LEAFLETS PROMISING TO VISIT US, AND
OTHERS NOT. AT THE SAME TIME HOWEVER I ALSO
NOTICED THAT THERE WERE SOME YOUTHS, WHO WERE
A LITTLE TOO NOISY TO SAY THE LEAST; OFTEN THE
POLICE CARS WOULD STOP TO TALK WITH THEM, AND
HAVING SPOKEN WITH THEM ONCE, AN OFFICER HAD
ADVICED ME THAT IT WAS BEST NOT TO APPROACH
THEM. OF COURSE I ALWAYS TRIED TO BE DISCERNING
AND PRUDENT, BUT I ALSO HAD TO DO MY JOB AND THEY
NEEDED GOD TOO.

I PREFERED AND I STILL DO, TO EVANGELISE IN THE OPEN
AIR, RATHER THAN GOING FROM HOUSE TO HOUSE,
THOUGH ONCE OR TWICE I RESOLVED TO KNOCK ON
SOME OF THE DOORS OF ONE OF THE ESTATES THERE.
THOUGH SOME WERE FRIENDLY, SOME WERE NOT KEEN
TO OPEN THE DOOR EITHER, LIKE A YOUNG WOMAN
WHO KEPT INSIDE HER FLAT AND ONLY OPENED THE
DOOR JUST ABOUT 15 CM. WIDE! THE TRUTH WAS THAT
SOME PEOPLE WERE LIVING IN AN ATMOSPHERE OF

FEAR! AND ONCE I EVEN EYE WITNESSED TO A YOUNG PERSON USING A GOLF METAL CLUB, SMASHING WITH IT THE DOOR AND I THINK THE WINDOW TOO OF HIS NEXT DOOR NEIGHBOUR IN THE ESTATE.

ALSO, UNLIKE JESUS, I TEND TO KEEP AWAY FROM CROWD AND I TEND TO APPROACH AND MINISTER TO ONE OR TWO PEOPLE AT THE TIME. HOWEVER AT LEAST ONCE, AS I WAS WITNESSING TO ONE OR TWO YOUNG PEOPLE, PRETTY SOON A SMALL GROUP OF THEM OF ABOUT MAYBE TEN TO FIFTEEN WAS GATHERED AROUND ME. I DID ENJOY TALKING TO THEM, AND SOME OF THEM WERE KEEN IN LISTENING AND KNEW ALSO OUR CHURCH VENUE WICH WAS IN FACT A YOUTH CENTRE.

I DID NOT LIKE THE FACT THAT SOME OF THESE WERE MOCKING, AND ONE AT LEAST STARTING TO SMACK ME ON MY HEAD IN A "PROVOKING AND UGLY PLAYFUL" WAY. IN AN OTHER OCCASION I THINK TWO YOUNG PEOPLE INSTIGATED THEIR DOGS AGAINST ME; ONE OF WICH AS I WAS TALKING WITH THEM WOULD BE JUMPING ON MY BACK. NOW WE DO NOT NEED TO BE PROPHETS TO UNDERSTAND, THAT WHEN THINGS LIKE THESE HAPPEN TO A 45 YEARS OLD MAN BY 15-17 YEARS OLDS, JUST FOR TRYING TO HAVE A TOLLERANT, RESPECTFUL AND PEACEFUL CHAT, AND UNFORTUNATELY MUCH WORST THAN THESE THINGS ARE HAPPENING IN LONDON EVEN TO OLDER PEOPLE TOO, SOME THINGS ARE GOING SERIOUSLY WRONG IN OUR SOCIETY!!! ANYHOW IN HISTORY THE CHURCH HAS ALWAYS BEEN PAYING A PRICE FOR SERVING GOD. A FEW

DAYS AGO' I HEARD A CATHOLIC PRIEST SAYING THAT JUST IN THER LAST CENTURY ABOUT 50 MILLIONS CHRISTIANS HAVE BEEN KILLED FOR THEIR FAITH.

BY THE WAY TOWARDS THE END OF MY SEVEN YEARS TERM WITH THIS CHURCH AND EVANGELISTIC ACTIVITY, I THINK THAT SOMEHOW, THOUGH I AM BEING A LITTLE IRONIC, I RECIEVED A KIND OF MEDAL TOO. BASICALLY A FEW TIMES I WAS ALSO ENCOURAGING SOME PEOPLE WHO WERE INVOLVED IN GAMBLING PEHAPS A LTTLE TO MUCH; INDEED ONE TOLD ME THAT HE HAD LOST ALMOST A MILLION POUNDS, AS HE WAS NOT ABLE TO CONTROL HIMSELF IN THIS ACTIVITY; I CERTAINLY TRIED TO HELP HIM, AND I HOPE OUR CHAT DID SO, THOUGH I REMEMBER HIM TO BE QUITE A DIFFICULT PERSON TO TALK TO. WELL IT HAPPENED THAT I WAS STANDING OUTSIDE, NOT FAR FROM THIS PARTICULAR BETTING SHOP, SUDDENLY, I THINK FROM ABOVE THE ONE FLOOR BUILDING NEXT TO THE BETTING SHOP, I WAS HIT RIGHT ON MY CHEST WITH AN EGG WHICH SPLASHED ON ME. I MAY SOUND SILLY TO YOU, BUT I WAS AND I AM STILL PROUD OF IT [LUKE 6: 22]. AFTER WASHING I CONTINUE TO MEET AND TO EVANGELISE PEOPLE IN THE MAIN ROADS.

NOW I AM GOING TO TELL YOU THE MOST INTERESTING DETAIL PERHAPS IN THIS PASSAGE BEING THE MAIN REASON FOR WHICH I AM WRITING IT. ONE EVENING, AS IT WAS NORMALLY MY CUSTOM TO BE THERE IN THE

EVENING, I WAS AGAIN IN THE MAIN ROAD LOOKING FOR PEOPLE THAT I COULD HELP WITH THE GOSPEL, SUDDENLY I SPOTTED ON MY RIGHT WALKING ALONG THE SHOPS, THE SAME YOUNG MAN WHO LOOKED A BIT OF A TROUBLE MAKER AND HAD SLAPPED ME SOME MONTHS EARLIER ME. HE WAS WALKING FAST, FOCUSED WITH HIS HEAD DOWN AND A LITTLE BENT; BUT THOUGH NONE OF HIS FRIENDS WERE WITH HIM, I JUST ABOUT MANAGED TO SEE THAT HE WAS IN FACT NOT ALONE! BUT AN EVIL SPIRIT WAS OVERSHADOWING HIM AND GOING ALONG WITH HIM. THE PITCURE THAT I REMEMBER VERY CLEARLY AS STILL FIXED IN MY MIND, IS THAT THAT SPIRIT WAS NOT PASSIVE AND NEITHER WAS HE SATISFIED IN KEEPING COMPANY TO THE YOUTH. ON THE CONTRARY HE LOOKED AS HE WAS LIKE TRYING TO INFLUENCE AND PROMPT THE YOUTH TO DO WRONG AND EVIL THINGS. IT WAS AS THAT DEMON WAS TRYING TO MENTOR AND FATHER THIS YOUNG MAN WITH A WRONG GOSPEL/INSTRUCTIONS. HE WAS CERTAINLY THERE FOR HIM!!! BUT NOT FOR GOOD, IN FACT FOR WICKEDNESS!!!

BASICALLY WE MUST BE AWARE THAT WE ARE AT WAR, LIKE JESUS WAS IN HIS MINISTRY!

PLEASE BE FREE TO MAKE YOUR OWN COMMENTS ON THIS, AS YOU KNOW IN THE SCRIPTURE VARIOUS DEMONIC ACTIVITIES INVOLVED PARTNERING WITH PEOPLE TOO [MARK 5 ; ACTS 5:3; 8: 9-13]. BUT THE

GOOD AND CONTRARY MODEL PER EXELLENCE TO THE DEMONIC JUST MENTIONED ABOVE, IS SEEN IN JESUS ACCOMPANIED AND ANOINTED BY THE HOLY SPIRIT, TO DO THE WILL OF THE FATHER DOING GOOD EVERY WHERE HE WENT AS ACTS 10: 38 TELLS US: < "HOW GOD ANOINTED JUSUS OF NAZARETH WITH THE HOLY SPIRIT AND WITH POWER, WHO WENT ABOUT DOING GOOD AND HEALING ALL WHO WERE OPPRESSED BY THE DEVIL, FOR GOD WAS WITH HIM. >

THE LEAST THAT WE CAN SAY IS THAT YOUNG PEOPLE IN OUR SOCIETIES NEED DISCEPLES MAKING MENTORS TO PROVIDE THEM WITH TRUE VALUES AND DIRECTIONS IN LINE WITH THE WILLL OF GOD. THUS IT IS VERY POSITIVE AND IMPORTANT THAT IN ALL CHURCHES, SUCH AS MINE TOO, WE PROVIDE THE YOUTHS AS WELL ALL MEMBERS: 1] WITH BOTH SMALL COURSES OPPORTUNITIES TO GROW IN CHRISTIAN KNOWLEDGE AND UNDERSTANDING, IN LEADERSHIP ABILITIES, AND 2] WITH SMALL GROUPS/CELLS/PASTORATES WHEREBY YOUNGER CHRISTIANS CAN LEARN FROM MORE EXPERIENCED; IN THESE GROUPS ALSO ALL FIND FELLOSHIP, ACCOUNTABILITY AND SUPPORTIVE FRIENDSHIP, LIKE IN A SMALL FAMILY CONTEXT, HELPING ONE ANOTHER TO BE EDIFIED IN THE LORD, AND TO BRING HIM MORE FRUIT AND GLORY, AMEN! IN FACT WE CAN SEE THAT BEARING OF FRUIT IS GOD'S REAL DESIRE FOR US AS JOHN 15:8 CLEARLY SHOWS US: < BY THIS MY FATHER IS GLORIFIED,

THAT YOU BEAR MUCH FRUIT; SO YOU WILL BE MY
DISCEPLES. >

****

I AM GOING TO TELL YOU NOW OF A PECULIAR, TO SAY
THE LEAST, EXPERIENCE OF MINE WHICH HAPPENED TO
ME HERE IN LONDON PERHAPS IN 1995. YOU ARE
ALREADY FAMILIAR WITH THE FACT THAT I WAS
BEFRIENDING AN IRANIAN FAMILY AND IN PARTICULAR
THIS WIDOW WHO ALSO SUFFERED FROM DEPRESSION [I
WOULD RATHER SAY LACK OF GOD AND FULFILMENT
OF GODLY ACTIVITIES, IN HER CASE AND IN MANY
OTHERS, AS JESUS CAME TO GIVE US LIFE
IN ABUNDANCE]. AND SO I WAS DOING MY BEST DO LEAD
THEM TO CHRIST, IN SPEAKING TO THEM, AS A MODEL
EXAMPLE, HELPING THEM AND PRAYING FOR THEM. HER
SISTER WAS DUE TO COME FROM AUSTRALIA TO VISIT
HER, AND THEY HAD INVITED ME ALSO TO MEET HER. THE
SISTER WAS MARRIED IN AUSTRALIA. UNFORTUNATELY I
THINK THE INTENTION OF HER SISTER WAS RATHER
DIFFERENT FROM A CHURCH CONTEX!

WELL IT HAPPENED THAT, BEING QUITE ZELOUS AND
PASSIONATE, I HAD DECIDED TO VISIT A LARGE NON-
CHRISTIAN INSTITUTION,"TO SEE WHAT WAS HAPPENING
THERE "BEFORE GOING TO MEET MY FRIENDS. AS I HAVE
ALREADY TOLD YOU, I AM QUITE TOLLERANT AND
RESPECTFUL TOWARDS OTHER PEOPLE' FREEDOM OF

BELIEFS. I ALSO MAKE A DIFFERENCE BETWEEN PEOPLE AND THEIR BELIEFS, AS IN FACT WE ARE CALLED TO LOVE ALL, AS EVEN JESUS GAVE HIMSELF FOR ALL BECAUSE OF HIS LOVE TOWARDS THE WORLD; THUS WE CAN LOVE ALL PEOPLE WHILE AT THE SAME TIME WE CAN DISAGREE WITH SOME OF THEIR BELIEFS, AND ENCOURAGE THEM TO CHANGE THEIR MINDS AND CONSIDER AND ACCEPT THE TRUTH IN CHRIST JESUS AND HIS WORD [MARK 1:14; JOHN 3:16]!

IN FACT AT THE SAME TIME, OUR MAIN AIM IS ALSO TO BE FAITHFUL TO THE LORD, WHO ALSO IS FAITHFUL IN HELPING US OVERCOMING OUR WEAKNESSES. WHAT IS ENCOURAGING FOR US IS THAT THE SCRIPTURES TEACH US THAT THOUGH WE LIVE IN THE FLESH, WE CAN AND ARE TO WALK IN THE SPIRIT (GAL. 5:21).

ANYWAY I WAS CURIOUS AND I MADE MY WAY TO VISIT THIS PLACE. IT WAS QUITE A LARGE BUILDING WITH A VERY SPACIOUS HALL FOR PEOPLE TO PRAY THERE. I DO NOT REMEMBER WHICH DAY IT WAS BUT THERE WERE A FEW DEVOTEES PRAYING. WELL I MUST HAVE HAD A LOOK AROUND, MAYBE THERE WAS A BOOKSHOOP TOO, PROBABLY I MUST HAVE GREETED SOME PEOPLE THERE ALSO. IT HAPPENED HOWEVER THAT I NEEDED TO USE THE TOILETS, AND I AM QUITE GLAD THAT I DID, AND YOU WILL SOON UNDERSTAND WHY.

I CANNOT REMEMBER EXCATLY MY PRECISE
MOVEMENTS, AND IT IS NOT THAT IMPORTANT THAT I
DO. WELL I DID ENTER THE TOILETTES, AND AS I WAS
LOOKING AROUND OBSERVING THAT THESE LOOKED
RATHER DIFFERENT FROM OUR USUAL EUROPEAN ONES,
SUDDENLY I EXPERIENCED SOMETHING VERY
INTERESTING. BY THE WAY I MUST HAVE BEEN AGAING "
IN THE SPIRIT ", OR UNDER THE INFLUNCE OR THE HOLY
SPIRIT ANYWAY, THOUGH I DID NOT KNOW IT AS I WAS
GOING THROUGH JUST THE BIGINNING STAGE OF
MY EXPERIENCES OF THE KINGDOM OF GOD AND OF THE
KINGDOM OF DARKNESS. WHAT HAPPENED THEN IS THAT
I STARTED TO SMELL A TERRIBLE STENCH OF
EXCREMENTS ABOVE ME, REALLY QUITE A LARGE
QUANTITY OF IT; IT WAS ALMOST LIKE IF THERE WAS AN
INVISIBLE STINKING CLOUD AROUND AND ABOVE ME,
THOUGH I ONLY SMELLED AND I SAW NOTHING AT ALL
THEN.

AT THAT MOMENT I THOUGH IT MUST HAVE BEEN
PERHAPS BECAUSE OF THE TOILETS BEING DIRTY, OR
MAYBE THE UNDERNEATH SEWAGES HAD NOT BEING
CLEANED WELL.

DESPITE FELING A BIT PUZZLED AND DOUBTFUL, REALLY I
HAD NO OTHER EXPLANATIONS, AS IN FACT AFTER
I REALIZED THAT THE PLACE WAS ACTUALLY CLEAN.
ANYHOW SLOWLY SLOWLY, AND CONTINUING TO
OBSERVE THE SURROUNDINGS, I BEGAN MY WAY OUT
AND TOWARDS MY FRIENDS' HOUSE. I THINK I MUST
HAVE BEEN A FEW MINUTES LATE FOR MY APPOINTMENT

WITH MY FRIEND AND HER SISTER, AND HAVING REACHED HER HOUSE, THERE WAS HER SISTER. SHE MUST HAVE BEEN 50-55 YEARS OLD, I GREETED HER, BY THE WAY I WAS STILL IN THE SPIRIT, I NOTICED THAT HER DRESS WAS SHOWING A PIECE OF HER RED BRA, SOMETHING THAT I DISLIKED,THEN I LOOKED AT HER STRAIGHT IN HER EYES, AND NONE OF US NEITHER CARED NOR WAS ANY OF US IMPRESSED WITH EACH OTHER. THEN SHE SAYED SOMETHING TO HER SISTER AND LEFT THE HOUSE.

TIME WENT BY I GOT TO KNOW THAT SHE OWNED SOME FLATS HERE IN LONDON AND THAT WITH HER HUSBAND HAD LOST A BUSINESS DEAL WORTH MANY MILLIONS OF AUSTRALIAN DOLLARS, AND SHE DID NOT CARE LESS; IN FACT BOTH HER AND HER SISTER [MY FRIEND], WERE FROM AN ARISTOCRATIC FAMILY IN IRAN. I WAS ALSO INVITED TO GO TO RUSSIA WITH HER, AND HAVING KINDLY EXPLAINED TO HER THAT I HAD NO TIME, SHE REPLIED TO ME THAT SHE WOULD MAKE TIME FOR ME. I CERTAINLY WAS MORE THAN HAPPY NOT TO GO WITH HER!

IT IS SAD BUT THIS IS THE REALITY FOR ALL PEOPLE IRRESPECTIVE TO WHERE THEY COME FROM; WHAT I MEAN IS THAT IT IS NOT EASY AT ALL TO DO GOD'S WORK ANYWHERE, BECAUSE ALSO OF OUR SPIRITUAL ENEMY.

NOW IT WAS ONLY A FEW MONTHS AFTER THAT
SOMETHING OCCURED TO ME OUSIDE MY LONDON
ACCOMODATION, THAT RECONNECTED MY MEMORY TO
THE EXPEREINCE I HAD IN THAT PARTICULAR RELIGIOUS
INSTITUTION HERE IN LONDON, JUST MENTIONED
ABOVE.

I WAS LIVING IN NORTH LONDON, IN THE KILBURN AREA
TO BE MORE PRECISE. THE HOUSE HAD A GARDEN, AND
IT WAS MADE UP ALL BY BEDSITS; I THINK THERE WERE
ABOUT NINE ROOMS AND WITH NINE MEN IN THEM, NOT
A SINGULAR WOMAN THERE, IT WAS LIKE A MONASTERY
IRONACLY SPEAKING; THE OWNERS WERE JEWISH. AS
USUALLY ONE MORNING I MADE MY WAY OUT OF MY
HOUSE, AND STRAIGHTAWAY, TO MY SURPRISE, I BEGAN
TO SMELL A TERIBLE STENCH OF EXCREMENTS ALL
AROUND ME, QUITE IN ABUNDANCE IN THE AIR, NOT IN A
NORMAL WAY.

NOT KNOWING ANY BETTER, I STARTED TO LOOK
AROUND ON THE FLOOR FOR POSSIBLE DOG'S
"DROPPINGS ". TO MY SURPRISE I COULD NOT FIND ANY.
FEELING VERY PUZLED AGAING, I BEGAN TO WALK ALONG
THE STREET ON THE PAVEMENT TOWARDS MY BUS
STOP, TO CATCH ONE OF MY USUAL BUSES TO TAKE ME
TO CENTRAL LONDON. I DO NOT KNOW WHAT BUT
SOMETHING MADE ME TURN MY HEAD AROUND AND
LOOK BACK. PLEASE DO KNOW THAT IT WAS IN THIS
PERIOD THAT I HAD BEGAN TO ATTEND BIBLE COLLEGE
TO TAKE MY FIRST CERTIFICATE IN CHRISTIAN MINISTRY,

THUS GRADUALLY INCREASING MY KNOWLEGE ALSO IN
THE SUBJECT OF "KNOWING YOUR ENEMY, SATAN ".

NOW AS I LOOKED BEHIND ME, WHAT I SAW WAS
SOMETHING THAT CAUGHT MY EYE STRAIGHTAWAY.
BEHIND ME WAS A MAN WALKING A LARGE DOG THAT
LOOKED LIKE A GERMAN SHEPERD; THIS MAN DID NOT
LOOK CLEAN IN HIS CLOTHES OR IN HIS APPEERENCE. I
FELT THERE WAS SOMETHING SINISTER ABOUT HIM, AND
HE ALSO WORE LARGE DARK GLASSES, AND SMILED AT
ME IN A RATHER BAD WAY. THEN I REALIZED THAT THE
MAN MUST HAVE BEEN A SATANIST OR SOMEHOW
INVOLVED IN THE OCCULTIC WORLD. THIS ALSO
EXPLAINED TO ME THE REASON FOR THAT TERRIBLE
STENCH IN SUCH A LARGE QUANTITY AND FOR NO
PHYSICAL NATURAL REASON BOTH IN THIS OCCASION AS
WELL AS IN THAT PARTICULAR NON-CHRISTIAN
RELIGIOUS INSTITUTION A FEW MONTHS EARLIER.

PLEASE NOTE AGAIN THAT THE MAIN PURPOSE OF THE
DEVIL IS TO DECIEVE PEOPLE AND SEPARATE THEM FROM
GOD AND THEMSELVES, THROUGH ANY MEANS POSSIBLE
TO HIM, WHETHER INFLUENCING MAN IN WORDS,
ACTIONS, THOUGHTS, OR BELIEFS, AS WE CAN OBSERVE
IN THE FOUNDATIONAL PASSAGE OF GEN. 3; OF WHICH V.
4-5 READ: < THEN THE SERPENT SAID TO THE WOMAN,
"YOU WILL NOT SURELY DYE."FOR GOD KNOWS THAT IN

THE DAY YOU EAT OF IT YOUR EYES WILL BE OPENED, AND YOU WILL BE LIKE GOD, KNOWING GOOD AND EVIL."
>

BASICALLY THE HOLY SPIRIT AGAIN, SINCE I WAS AND STILL AM ACTIVE IN DOING HIS WORK, LET ME TAP IN HIS POWER, I THINK IN BOTH THIS CASES IN THE GIFT OF DISCERNMENT [1 COR. 12:10]; IN THIS WAY THAT I COULD SEE AND UNDERSTAND SPIRITUAL SOURCES AND THEIR AGENDAS. IT IS GOD EQUIPPING US WITH ALL KIND OF GIFTS TO DO HIS WORK, NOT FOR SELF AND SELFISH INTERESTS BUT FOR THE COMMON GOOD AND PROFIT OF ALL [1 COR. 12:1-7].

MOST INTERESTINGLY WE KONW THAT DEMONS ARE REFERED TO BY JESUS AS "UNCLEAN SPIRITS ", ALSO IN THE OLD TESTAMENT THE DEVIL WAS OFTEN REFERED TO AS THE PRINCE OF THE FILTH, OR THE LORD OF THE FLIES [2 KINGS 1:2; MATTH. 12:27; 1 TIM. 4: 1-5]. BUT LET US LOOK AT MARK 9:25 TOGETHER: WHEN JESUS SAW THAT THE PEOPLE CAME RUNNING TOGETHER, HE REBUKED THE UNCLEAN SPIRIT, SAYING TO IT: "DEATH AND DUMB SPIRIT, I COMMAND YOU, COME OUT OF HIM AND ENTER HIM NO MORE!" >

IT IS OBVIOUS THAT IF THEY ARE UNCLEAN THEY MUST ALSO SMELL, BUT I PREFER NOT TO RISK SPECULATING; CERTAINLY FILTH AND FLIES NEITHER DO THEY LOOK PLEASANT NOR DO THEY SMELL NICE!

SADLY TO SAY THIS LADY FRIEND OF MINE BECAME WORSE AND WORSE IN HER HEALTH AND MAYBE SPIRITUALLY TOO. I HAD VISITED A FEW TIMES IN HER HOME, AND MY ANALYSIS OF HER LIFE WAS THAT MOSTLY, HER MISSION WAS HER BED AND HER TELEVISION, CONTRARY TO WHAT WE SEE IN THE SCRIPTURES FOR US.

ONE DAY COMING INTO HER FLAT, I SAT IN HER BEDROOM TO KEEP HER SOME COMPANY; HER ROOM WAS FILLED WITH FLIES, PERHAPS THIRTY OR SO; LUCKILY THE DOOR WAS OPEN TO THE BALCONY ON WHICH FLOOR THERE WAS LEFT MUCH OF HER PET DOG'S EXCREMENTS. TO MY SURPRISE AS I SAT THERE FACING HER AND HER BED, AS SHE USED TO WATCH TV FROM HER BED, THE FLIES LEFT; MAYBE ONLY ONE, TWO OR THREE WERE LEFT WHILE I WAS THERE, PRAISE GOD!

DESPITE TILL TODAY I DO NOT KNOW THE TRUTH, I HEARD THAT A FEW YEARS LATER SHE COMMITTED SUICIDE WITH AN OVERDOSE OF SOME OF HER USUAL MEDICATIONS. NOT SURE OF THE CIRCUMSTANCES OF HER LAST MINUTES, EVEN TODAY IT IS MY HOPE THAT SHE MET THE SAVIOR BEFORE SHE LEFT THIS WORLD. I HOPE THAT FOR HER CONFORT HER GROWN UP CHILDREN MUST HAVE BEEN WITH HER IN THOSE MOMENTS, AND IN PRAYER WITH YOU, THAT THESE WILL GROW AND LIVE WITH A GOOD RELATIONSHIP WITH OUR LORD JESUS, AMEN .

******

WHAT FOLLOW NEXT IS A VERY BRIEF STORY THAT
HAPPENED TO ME RIGHT AT THE BEGINNING OF MY
CHRISTIAN LIFE FILLED WITH THE HOLY SPIRIT, PERHAPS
IN 94 OR 95. ALSO IT IS SOMETHING THAT EVEN TODAY I
DO NOT FULLY UNDERSTAND, NEITHER AM I ABLE TO
FIND A 100% SATISFYING ANSWER FROM THE
SCRIPTURES. THOUGH I HAVE A BURDEN TO TALK ABOUT
IT, I WILL NOT BE ABLE TO MAKE ANY REAL COMPLETE
CONCLUSIONS, AND NEITHER WILL I EXPECT YOU TO
BELIEVE IT, UNLESS YOUR UNDERSTANDING OF THE
SCRIPTURES ALLOW YOU TO DO SO!

NOW IN THAT TIME I WAS LOOKING FOR
ACCOMODATION AND IT HAPPENED THAT I CAME
ACROSS A NOTICE BY AN ITALIAN LADY; THOUGH HER
ACCOMODATION WAS NOT SUITABLE FOR ME, WE
REMAINED IN TOUCH AND, AS I HAVE ALREADY
MENTIONED EARLIER IN THIS BOOK, WE BECAME
FRIENDS. IT WAS THIS LADY WHO HAD INTRODUCED ME
TO THE IRANIAN LADY, WHOM I HAVE JUST MENTIONED
ABOVE. UNFORTUNATELY THOUGH SHE CAME FROM A
RELIGIOUS CATHOLIC BACKGROUND, SHE WAS NOT
LEADING A REALLY COMMITTED CHRISTIAN LIFE, AND
EVEN TODAY I DO NOT WHETHER SHE IS A REAL BELIEVER
OR JUST A NOMINAL ONE.

ANYHOW AT TIMES I USED TO GO OUT WITH HER AND EVEN VISIT HER HOUSE; SHE ALSO CAME TO CHURCH WITH ME AT LEAST TWICE, AND I GOT TO KNOW PART OF HER FAMILY TOO.

CLEARLY HER LIFE AND HISTORY AS WELL AS OURS CAN ONLY TRULY BE SIGNIFICANT IN GOD OUR SAVIOUR; HOWEVER GOD IS SO MERCIFUL THAT HE EVEN USES ANYONE TO SHAPE THE HISTORY OF THE WORLD.

MOVING ON WITH THIS STORY OF MINE, THE SINISTER EXPERIENCE THAT HAPPENED TO ME IN THIS LITTLE ACCOUNT ACTUALLY OCCURED IN HER FLAT, DURING ONE OF MY VISITS TO HER. BEING MUCH YOUNGER AND LESS EXPERIENCED I SHOULD HAVE KEPT A WIDER DISTANCE FROM HER AND HER FRIENDS, BUT SADLY NONE IS BORN PERFECT, NOR CAN HE LIVES A PERFECT CHRISTIAN LIFE. SO I WAS TRYING TO EVANGELISE HER AND HER FRIENDS, BUT AT THE SAME TIME I ALSO WAS SOCIALISING WITH THEM TO MY RISK AND LOSS TOO. I DO NOT REMEMENBER EXCATLY THE DETAILS OF THAT EVENING OR AFTERNOON, BUT THERE I WAS IN HER FLAT WITH HER AND PERHAPS WITH TWO OR THREE OF HER FRIENDS/FAMILY MEMBERS. I REMEMBER THAT AT TIME WE USED TO PLAY CARDS, BUT THIS TIME I THINK WE WERE JUST TALKING OR WATCHING TV, OR PERHAPS I WAS PREACHING OR READING THE BIBLE TO HER/THEM.

WHATEVER WE WERE DOING IS NOT CLEAR TO ME NOW AND IT IS NOT TOO IMPORTANT EITHER. SUDDENLY AS I WAS SITTING THERE, I FELT A STRONG PAIN RIGHT ABOVE ME. I DID NOT SEE NOR HEAR ANYTHING AROUND ME, I JUST FELT THIS CLEAR PAIN ABOVE MY HEAD, BUT NOT IN MY HEAD. IT WAS LIKE IF SOMEONE, I GUESS THE DEVIL, HAD BEEN SAWING ME ABOVE MY HEAD, MAKING ME FEEL PAINFUL FOR 2 OR 3 SECONDS; AND THAT IS ALL THAT HAPPENED.

I DID FEEL A BIT SCARED AND SHOCKED THAT THE FOLLOWING WEEK IN CHURCH I HAD TO PRAY WITH SOMEONE ABOUT IT, AT LEAST FOR CONFORT, REASSURANCE AND STRENGTH.

WITHOUT DOUBT IT MUST HAVE BEEN A DEMONIC ATTACK AGAINST ME; PROBABLY WHAT THE DEVIL WAS SAYING WAS THAT I WAS NOT TO INTERFERE WITH THOSE PEOPLE AND IN THAT PLACE AS IT WAS UNDER HIS INFLUENCE, AND I WAS NOT TO TAKE IT ALL AWAY FROM HIM.

I DO NOT HAVE A PROBLEM IN BELIEVING THIS, AS THIS IS THE ENEMY'S STRATEGY ANYWAY, AND ALL THESE PEOPLE WERE LIVING IN SIN SADLY [MATTH. 12:27-29]. OBVIOUSLY THE DEVIL DOES NOT LIKE US OR OUR WORK, BUT WE MUST TAKE ADVANTAGE OF THE HARVEST THAT THE LORD BRINGS TO OUR WAY.

BUT WHAT I DO NOT UNDERSTAND IS THE DETAILS OF HIS ATTACK ON ME: 1- WHERE DID IT HURT ME? WHAT WAS IT ON MY HEAD? DO WE HAVE A SPIRITUAL LINE ABOVE OUR HEAD THAT CONNECTS US TO GOD AND HEAVEN? AND WAS HE TRYING TO SAW/SEVERE/CUT IT, IN ORDER TO UNDERMINE OR HURT MY RELATIONSHIP AND INTERCESSORY POSITION AND POWER BEFORE AND WITH GOD?

COULD POSSIBLY THE SILVER CORD MENTIONED HERE BY ECCLESIASTES 12:6 CONTRIBUTE IN UNDERSTANDING THIS ISSUE? DIFFICULT TO SAY, AS THIS PASSAGE COULD JUST REFER TO VARIOUS WAYS THROUGH WHICH THE WRITER IS PITCURING DEATH. I WANT TO FURTHER COMMENT THAT THE MUST BE A LINK BETWEEN US HERE AND US IN THE HEAVENLY REALM, SINCE AS THE APOSTLE PAUL PUTS IT IN EPHES. 2:5-6, WE ARE ASO...: < EVEN WHEN WE WERE DEAD IN TRESPASSES, MADE US ALIVE TOGETHER WITH CHRIST (BY GRACE YOU HAVE BEEN SAVED), AND RAISED US UP TOGETHER, AND MADE US SIT TOGETHER IN THE HEAVENLY PLACES IN CHRIST JESUS. >

FOR SURE, HOWEVER WE CERTAINLY KNOW THAT DEMONS ARE LYING, DECIEVING, ACCUSING, VIOLENT SPIRITS AND ROBBERS TOO [JOHN 8:44; REV. 16:14; 20:8]. NO WANDER ALSO WHY EVEN PRESENTLY MUCH VIDEOS AND TV PROGRAMS, AS WELL AS EVENTS IN WORLD AFFAIRS AND IN LIFE IN OUR COMMUNITIES ARE SO RICH AND FERTILE WITH IMMORALITY AND VIOLENCE. ALL VERY WELL RESEMBLING THE LIFE AS THE OLD TESTAMENT PITCURES IT TO US, STARTING FROM THE

FIRST BROTHERS TO FINISH WITH THE VARIOUS PAGAN GODS AND WARS THROUGHOUT THE OLD TESTAMENT; SINCE USUALLY THESE WERE PAGAN GODS OF SEXUAL FERTILITY AND WAR.

ANYHOW AFTER THAT DAY I BECAME MORE CAUTIOUS IN GOING TO HER FLAT LESS OFTEN, TO AVOID UNHEALTHY INVITATIONS TOO. DESPITE THIS KIND OF STRANGE EVENT, I DID NOT SUFFER MUCH, AND MY CHRISTIAN APOSTOLIC LIFE CONTINUED AS NORMALLY AND AS SUPERNATURALLY AS USUALLY IN THE CONFIDENCE OF THE HOLY SPIRIT. FOR WE NEED TO CONTINUE TO HELP ALL, DESPITE DIFFERENT BELIEFS.

I CANNOT BUT CONCLUDE THIS SMALL PASSAGE BY THANKING THE LORD FOR HIS CONTINUOUS PRAYERS IN PROTECTING US FROM THE EVIL ONE AS IN LUKE 11:1-4 AND JOHN 17. AND WE CAN LIVE WITH THIS CONFIDENCE BECAUSE HEBR 7:25 TELLS THAT: < THEREFORE HE IS ALSO ABLE TO SAVE TO THE UTTERMOST THOSE WHO COME TO GOD THROUGH HIM, SINCE HE ALWAYS LIVES TO MAKE INTERCESSION FOR THEM. > AMEN.

****

PLEASE NOTE THAT THIS STORY IS DIFFERENT FROM ALL THE REST OF THIS BOOK, AND HAS NOT REALLY HAPPEND TO ME!

THIS ACCOUNT WHICH I AM ABOUT TO TALK TO YOU
NOW IS UNFORTUNATLY QUITE A SAD ONE, THAT ANY
FAMILY WOULD DREAD IT WOULD HAPPEN TO THEM;
ALSO USUALLY NO FAMILY WOULD BELIEVE IT WOULD
HAPPEN TO THEM EITHER. WELL IT DID HAPPEN TO A
FRIEND OF MINE, A PASTOR LIKE ME AND HIS FAMILY. IT
IS A SERIES OF EVENT THAT HAPPENED PEHAPS BETWEEN
3 TO 7 YEARS AGO'. THIS PASTOR IS IN LONDON AS A
MISSSIONARY AND ALL HIS FAMILY IS IN ITALY. FOR
SOMETIMES HIS SISTER SEEMED TO HAVE BEEN
SUFFERING FROM SOME KIND OF SPIRITUAL/MENTAL
ISSUES, SHE OFTEN USED TO SCREAM LOUDLY, AND
SOMETIMES TERRIBLY LOUDLY. SHE SEEMED TO BE FILLED
WITH BITTERNESS AND ANGER AGAINST OTHER PEOPLE.

SADLY THIS WAS NOT ALL, BUT SHE SEEMED TO BE
HOSTILE TOWARDS THE CHURCH TOO, PEHAPS
BECAUSE SHE HAD SOME BAD EXPERIENCES WITH SOME
CHURCH PEOPLE LIKE NUNS AND PRIESTS. THUS VERY
SADLY SHE WOULD NOT SHOW INTEREST TOWARDS GOD
EITHER, BUT ON THE CONTRARY SEEMED TO BE ALMOST
HOSTILE TO THIS GENERAL CONTEXT.

THOUGH AT TIMES SHE COULD REASON PERFECTELY
WELL, SHE WOULD OFTEN SPEAK TO HERSELF, IGNORING
OTHERS AROUND HER. EVEN MORE SADLY WAS THE FACT
THAT AS SHE REASONED WITH HER FAMILY SHE WOULD
EXPLAIN THAT SHE WAS CONVINCED THAT PEOPLE WERE
CONTROLLING HER, PERHAPS EVEN WITH MICROCHIPS;

THEREFORE SHE WAS EVEN VERY CAREFUL IN WHAT TO
DRINK IN HER VERY HOUSE, BEING SCARED THAT
SOMEONE WOULD POISON HER.

SO AT TIMES SHE COULD DO THINGS FAIRLY OK IN THE
HOME AND HELPING LOOKING AFTER THEIR OLD
MOTHER. AT OTHER TIMES HOWEVER, IT WAS VERY
HARD AND ALL THE FAMILY WOULD SUFFER, ESPECIALLY
ONE OF HER BROTHERS AND HER MOTHER LIVING THERE.
IN THIS ENTIRE SITUATION SHE WOULD REFUSE GETTING
MEDICATIONS. LIFE FOR A FEW YEARS WAS VERY HARD
INDEED FOR HER AND HER FAMILY. AT TIMES,
AND WEEKLY IN A CERTAIN STAGE, HER POOR BROTHER
WOULD HAVE TO SLEEP IN A HOTEL AFTER WORK AS SHE
WOULD LOCK HIM OUTSIDE; ONCE EVEN THIS HAPPENED
TO HER BROTHER PASTOR BEING THERE ON HOLIDAYS. AT
OTHER TIMES THE DOOR OF THE FLAT HAD TO BE KEPT
UNLOCKED DURING THE DAY AS SHE WOULD PUT
SUPERGLUE IN THE LOCK CAUSING IT TO BE USELESS!

IT WAS ALSO QUITE DIFFICULT FOR HER BROTHER
PASTOR LIVING IN LONDON, AS HE WOULD FEEL ALL THIS
IN A VERY INTENSE WAY TOO, KNOWING THAT ALSO IS
MOTHER WAS NOT LOOKED AFTER PROPERLY. EVEN
CALLING ON THE PHONE FROM LONDON IN THE HOPE TO
SPEAK TO HIS MOTHER, AT TIMES SHE WOULD NOT
ALLOW HIM AND PUT THE PHONE DOWN, OR CUT THE
CONVERSATION, OR OFTEN NOT EVEN PICK UP THE
PHONE, OR OFTEN NOT MAKING ANY SENSE ON THE

PHONE BY BEING QUITE, UNFRIENDLY, OR USELESS.
WHAT WAS EVEN WORSE IS THAT THERE WERE
RUMOURS THAT SHE WOULD GO OUT CARRYING A PAIR
OF LONG SCISSORS IN HER HANDBAG FOR SELF DEFENCE,
THOUGH THIS FEAR WAS JUT ALL IN HER MIND. IN THE
MIST OF ALL THIS SITUATION THIS PASTOR FRIEND OF
MINE TOLD ME THAT ONE MORNING AS HE WAS AWAKE,
IN HIS HOUSE IN LONDON, NEAR HIS BED, A DEMON
SPOKE TO HIM SAYING << THIS TIME I REALLY HAVE
HURTED HER >>. THE NATURE OF HIS VOICE WAS NASTY
AND VERY WICKED!

IN HIS ATTEMPT TO CONTACT HER AND HIS MOTHER
THAT DAY, HIS SISTER WAS VERY HOSTILE AND HE WAS
NOT ABLE TO COMMUNICATE WITH THEM AT ALL.

WELL I GUESS THE STORY COMES TO A PICK DURING HIS
NEXT HOLIDAY TO ITALY TO VISIT HIS FAMILY. THERE
THEY WERE IN THE SITTING ROOM HAVING DINNER;
SUDDENLY HIS SISTER GRABBED TWO TABLE KNIVES AND
SAYED SOMETHING LIKE THIS << COME ON WHO WANTS
TO PLAY NOW? >>. IT WAS SIMPLY ASTONISHING AND
SCARING!!!

DURING THOSE TEN DAYS OF HOLIDAYS THERE, THIS
PASTOR SAW THAT HIS SISTER WOULD WALK IN THE FLAT
WITH THAT LONG PAIR OF SCISSORS IN HER POCKETS; ON
SOME OCCASIONS SHE THREATENED BOTH HIM AND HIS
BROTHER, POINTING THE SCISSORS AND/OR A KNIFE TO
THEM. THE PROBLEM WAS ALSO THE FACT THAT SHE
WAS NOT SURE ABOUT THEIR IDENTITY, AS AT TIMES SHE

WAS PRESUMING THEY WERE STRANGERS THAT LOOKED
LIKE HIS BROTHERS!

CERTAINLY IT MUST HAVE BEEN A TERRIFYING VIEW TO
SEE THIS OLD MOTHER AT LEAST ONCE, BEING ASSISTED
BY HER DAUGHTER WITH ONE HAND HOLDING A PAIR OF
SCISSORS! I CAN ONLY COMMENT THAT THIS CAN ONLY
BE SOMETHING LIKE A PREVIEW OF HELL ITSELF!

THANKS GOD THAT, THOUGH DESPITE FEARS AND
VARIOUS RISKS, DECISIONS WERE MADE TO CONTACT
HER GP, A LOCAL PSYCHIATRIST, AND THE HEAD OF THE
POLICE THERE IN ORDER TO TREAT HER WITH
MEDICATIONS BY FORCE! WELL THE STORY GOES ON
THAT NOW SHE IS ON MEDICATIONS, AND SHE IS FEELING
AND BEHAVING FAIRLY WELL; SHE IS ALSO LOOKING
AFTER HER MOTHER MUCH BETTER, AND AT TIME SHE
HAS BEEN TAKEN UP VARIOUS COURSES TOO. I AM ALSO
GLAD TO HEAR THAT SHE IS ALSO GOING TO CHURCH
TOO.

SHE IS VERY WELL AWARE THAT SHE MUST NOT DROP
HER MEDICATIONS AS SHE WOULD GET SICK AGAIN.
MOREOVER SHE REGULARLY VISITS A SPECIALIST. I HAVE
BEEN TOLD BY THIS FRIEND OF MINE THAT SHE SUFFERS
FROM SOME KIND OF CHEMICAL IMBALANCE. I KNOW
THAT NOW SHE IS ACTIVE LOOKING FOR A JOB, BEING
MUCH BETTER. I AM SURE THAT, AS YOU READ THIS,
THAT YOU WILL AGREE IN PRAYER WITH ME, THAT SHE

WILL BE RESTORED TO A SUCCESFUL CAREER, AS SHE IS A VERY EDUCATED PERSON; IN ADDITION THAT SHE AND HER FAMILY SHALL WALK WITH GOD AND NEVER EXPERIENCE SUCH DRAMAS AGAIN, AMEN!

ANYHOW, VERY BRIEFLY I WOULD LIKE TO THANK GOD AND THESE DOCTORS AS THEY HAVE SUCCEEDED TO TREAT HER FAIRLY WELL. SECONDLY HOWEVER, I WOULD LIKE TO COMMENT AND SAY THAT I CAN CERTAINLY ACCEPT THAT IN THIS AND SOME OTHER CASES CHEMICAL IMBALANCE IS A FACT AND THUS MEDICATIONS MUST BE USED TO ENABLE A BALANCED OPERATION OF THE BRAIN. BUT I WOULD LIKE TO ADD THAT IN SOME CASES AS IN THIS TOO THERE IS A DEMONIC ELEMENT AT WORK ALSO.

I BELIEVE WITHOUT A SHADOW OF DOUBT THAT IN THIS CASE MUCH DAMAGE WAS DONE BY EVIL SPIRITS, WHO PERHAPS DID SO, ALSO AS REVENGE TO HER BROTHER WHO IS A PASTOR AND A PREACHER OF THE GOSPEL. ALSO SHE MAY HAVE OPENED DOORS TO DEMONIC PUNISHMENTS AS I WAS TOLD THAT AT SOME STAGES IN THE PAST, THIS LADY HAD DESPISED THE SCRIPTURES AND THE CHURCH, AS WELL AS BECAUSE OF THIS JUDGEMENTAL ATTITUDE, ANGER, BITTERNESS AND UNFORGIVENESS TOWARDS OTHERS. IN FACT PAUL CLEARLY WARNS US IN EPH. 4:25-32: <...DO NOT LET THE SUN GO DOWN ON YOUR WRATH. NOR GIVE PLACE TO THE DEVIL...LET NO CORRUPT WORD PROCEED OUT OF YOUR MOUTH, BUT WHAT IS GOOD FOR NECESSARY EDIFICATION, THAT IT MAY IMPART GRACE TO THE

HEARERS. AND DO NOT GRIEVE THE HOLY SPIRIT...LET ALL BITTERNESS, WRATH, ANGER, CLAMOR, AND EVIL SPEAKING BE PUT AWAY FROM YOU, WITH ALL MALICE. AND BE KIND TO ONE ANOTHER...>. AND IN JESUS' WORDS << ... FOR WHOEVER HAS, TO HIM MORE WILL BE GIVEN; AND WHOEVER DOES NOT HAVE, EVEN WHAT HE SEEMS TO HAVE WILL BE TAKEN AWAY FROM HIM >> [LUKE 8:18]. ANYHOW WE MUST CERTAINLY BE AWARE AND ALERT AS THIS SPIRITUAL ENEMY IS AGAINST US GOD'S CREATURES; BUT WE MUST ALSO REJOICE AS IN CHRIST WE HAVE OVERCOME HIM [JOHN 16:33; 1 JOHN 2: 13]!

******

FINALLY IN THIS CHAPTHER THE FOLLOWING STORY IS INSTEAD QUITE A RECENT ONE THAT HAPPENED TO ME ABOUT 2-3 YEARS AGO'. FOR SOME TIME I USED TO SEE IN A COFFE SHOP AN OLDER MAN AND A WOMAN, LOOKING ON THEIR SIXTEES/SEVENTEES AND THOUGH NOT TOO SURE, I HAD HEARD BEFORE MEETING EITHER OF THEM PERSONALLY, THAT THEY USED TO ATTEND SOME KIND OF SPIRITUALISTIC CHURCH WHERE THERE ARE PEOPLE ACTING AS MEDIUMS, TO BRING MESSAGES FROM THE DEAD TO THEIR LIVING RELATIVES. IT HAPPENED HOWEVER THAT PEHAPS 2-3 YEARS AFTERWARDS I HAD A CHAT WITH THIS LADY; SHE

CONFIRMED THAT THIS WAS THEIR PRACTISE: EVERY
SUNDAY TO GO TO THIS SPIRITUALISTIC CHURCH WITH
HER MAN FRIEND. I WAS ALSO READING THE SCRIPTURES
WHEN WE MET AND FROM THESE I SHOWED AND
EXPLAINED TO HER THAT WHAT SHE WAS DOING WAS
AGAINST GOD'S WORD AND THUS AGAINST GOD'S
BLESSINGS IN HER LIFE [DEUT. 18].

I WAS GLAD THAT SHE HAD EARS TO HEAR AND SHE
STARTED TO STOP GOING TO THIS PLACE AND BEGAN
EVEN TO COME TO OUR CHURCH MEETINGS, WHERE SHE
TOLD ME SHE PATICULARLY ENJOYED ITS MUSIC AND THE
SINGING. I ALSO KNOW THAT SHE WAS GREATFULT TO
GOD FOR THE MANY OTHER GOOD ACTIVITIES
HAPPENING THERE SUCH AS THE HEALINGS, THE
TEACHINGS, AND THE VARIOUS DEGREES OF FELOWSHIP
OFFERED BY THIS MINISTRY. IN FACT SHE JOINED ALSO A
CELL GROUP WITH OTHER WOMEN AND BEGAN SMALL
CHRISTIAN COURSES TO GROW MORE IN THE FAITH. THIS
LADY WAS AND IS A GREAT GRANDMOTHER, SEPARATE
FROM HER HUSBAND WHO HAS NOW CHILDREN FROM
AN OTHER WOMAN. THOUGH SHE WAS NOT IN VERY
GOOD RELATIONS WITH HER CHILDRENS, WITH GOD'S
GRACE SHE ALSO BEGAN TO IMPROVE HER RELATIONSHIP
WITH THEM. AT TIMES I HAVE BEEN MEETING FOR COFFE
WITH HER AND SHE TOLD ME THAT EVEN THIS EASTER
SHE WAS IN ONE OF HER SON'S HOUSE.

NOW AFTER FEW WEEKS I HAD MET HER, I LEARNED
FROM HER THAT SHE WAS A HOLDER AND THAT
BASICALLY HER FLAT WAS IN A MESS; SO LIFE FOR HER
AND HER CAT WAS A BIT DIFFICULT AT THE MOMENT. I
BELIEVE THAT IT WAS GOD WHO GAVE ME THE
STRENGHT SLOWLY SLOWLY, TO HELP HER CLEAR ALL THE
MESS FROM HER FLAT. YOU COULD HARDLY
WALK THROUGH IN THIS ONE BEDROOM FLAT, AS IT WAS
CROWDED WITH ALL KIND OF THINGS THAT SHE REALLY
NEEDED NOT: OLD FURNITURE, OLD CLOTHES, CLOTHES
MUCH BIGGER THAN HER SIZE, MUSICAL RECORDS,
VIDEOS, MANY KIND OF OBJECTS ON SHELVES AND ON
THE FLOOR TAKING VITAL SPACE, OLD AND BAD
MAGAZINES AND BOOKS, ETC..

SO I BEGAN WITH HER TO CLEAR THIS MESS; AND I THINK
IT TOOK US ABOUT 3 MONTHS TO DO SO. WITHOUT
COUNTING THE LARGE OLD FURNITURES THAT SHE
REPLACED WITH GOOD ONES, I BELIEVE THAT WE MUST
HAVE GOT RID OF ABOUT 50-60 FULL LARGE BLACK BACKS
OF THIS STAFF!

OBVIOUSLY I PRAYED ABOUT IT TOO, AND I KNEW THAT
THIS WAS IN GREAT PART DUE TO DEMONIC INFLUENCE
IN HER LIFE, DUE TO HER SINFUL LIFE STYLE THAT SHE
WAS LIVING. I ALSO ASKED THE LORD TO GIVE ME AN
ANSWER, AND TOUGH USUSALLY I DO NOT DREAM, ONE
NIGHT I HAD A DREAM AND I SAW LIKE A DIRTY AND
UGLY LOOKING MAN RUNNING AWAY FROM HER LIFE!

THIS REPRESENTED A DEMON FOR ME: BASICALLY SHE WAS BEING DELIVERED BOTH SPIRITUALLY AND PRACTICALLY IN HER FLAT! TO GOD'S GLORY SHE ALSO MANAGED TO PUT ON SOME WEIGHT AS WELL AS STARTED TO LIVE A BETTER LIFE CLOSE TO GOD AND WITH LESS DEPRESSION TOO.

THIS IS NOT ALL THAT I WANT TO TELL YOU.

SHE HAD BEEN 5 YEARS WITHOUT SEEING HER MOTHER WHO WAS LIVING BACK IN THE PORTUGHESE ISLAND OF MADEIRA. THE MOTHER WAS ABOUT 90 YEARS OLD, A GREAT, GREAT GRANDMOTHER! AND SO BECAUSE OF GOD'S FAVOUR I WAS ABLE TO TAKE HER THERE TO SEE HER MOTHER IN MADEIRA IN THE FOLLOWING YEAR. THE MOTHER WAS STILL HEALTHY ENOUGH TO GO OUT WITH US FOR SOMETIMES; BUT I FELT SAD THAT SHE, NOW A WIDOW, WAS LIVING ALONE IN THIS 3 BEDROOM HOUSE WITH 3 FLOORS; THE STAIRS ALSO WERE QUITE STEEP. WHAT MADE ME EVEN MORE SAD WAS THAT SHE WOULD KEEP ALL THE SHUTTERS OF THE HOUSE CLOSED, AND SO THERE WAS NOT MUCH LIGHT IN ALL HER HOUSE. ONE OF THE THINGS THAT I CARED TO DO THERE WAS TRYING TO HELP HER HAVE PASSION FOR THE WORD OF GOD AND SO TO READ IT, TO HELP HER TO FEEL BETTER TOO.

AGAIN HOWEVER SOMETHING STRANGE AND SINISTER HAPPENED TO ME THERE. ONE NIGHT AS I WAS RESTING EARLY IN THE MORNING, THOUGHTS WERE COMING TO ME, "SOME THINGS WERE STRESSING ME" [I THINK

PERHAPS "LITTLE DEMONS "], OR I WAS BEING
HARASSED BY THIS EVIL SPIRIT THAT I AM ABOUT TO
MENTION. ON THIS PLEASE TAKE GOOD NOTE OF MATTH.
9:36: < BUT WHEN HE SAW THE MULTITUDES, HE WAS
MOVED WITH COMPASSION FOR THEM, BECAUSE THEY
WERE WEARY {HARASSED} AND SCATTERED, LIKE SHEEP
HAVING NO SHEPERD. >

DISTURBING, ANNOYING AND STRESSING
THOUGHTS WERE COMING TO MY MIND AND
BOTHERING ME. I BEGAN TO BE MORE AWAKE AND
AWAKE, AND SUDDENLY A DEMON SPOKE TO ME
CLEARLY IN ENGLISH SAYING WITH A HARD AND
ARROGANT VOICE << AND YOU WHAT ARE YOU DOING
HERE? >>.

THIS DEMON SEEMED TO HAVE BEEN SURPRISED TO SEE
ME THERE. I FELT AS HE KNEW ABOUT ME AND SO WAS
SOMEHOW SURPRISED AND DISPLEASED TO SEE ME
THERE TOO; THUS HE WAS TRYING TO MESS HIM
AROUND IN THAT HOUSE. WITHOUT DOUBT I BELIEVE
THAT IT WAS HIS WORK TO PUT OFF THIS FRIEND'S
MOTHER FROM READING THE BIBLE AND GOING TO
CHURCH; ALSO FOR KEEPING HER IN THE DARK IN HER
HOUSE WITH ALL THE SHUTTERS CLOSED. IT WAS ALSO
PROBABLY ONE OF HIS WORK, THE DEATH OF THIS LADY'S
FATHER [THAT IS THE OLDER LADY'S FIRST HUSBAND],
WHEN SHE WAS STILL A BABY, THOUGH DIFFICULT TO SAY
FOR SURE IN THE LATTER CASE.

STILL WE KNOW THAT IT IS THE DEVIL WHO DESTROYS LIVES, FAMILIES AND COMMUNITIES, SOMETIMES WITH THE HELP OF MEN TOO [JOHN 10:10].

ANYHOW THAT WAS ALL AND IN THE MORNING I GOT UP AND SPEND AN OTHER DAY THERE AS USUSAL.

I THINK TO HAVE TOLD THIS STORY TO THIS LADY FRIEND OF MINE FOR HER OWN BENEFIT. DURING THIS WEAK, I HELPED HER TO VISIT SOME RELATIVES AND FRIENDS AND IT CERTAINLY WAS ALSO FOR ME A NICE HOLIDAY IN THIS BEAUTIFUL, THOUGH VULCANIC ISLAND. HERE IN PARTICULARLY I ENJOYED SEEING FOR THE FIRST TIME MANY BANANA TREES; I FOUND OF GREAT BEAUTY THE PAVEMENTS IN THE CAPITAL FUNCHAL AS MADE LIKE A MOSAIC WITH TINY BLACK AND WHITE STONES, PUT BY HANDS. THIS LATTER FEATURE REMINDED ME OF THE FUTURE GLORY OF THE NEW JERUSALEM WHICH WILL BE PAVED WITH GOLD TO THE GLORY OF GOD AS SHOWN IN REV. 21:21: < THE TWELVE GATES WERE TWELVE PEARLS: EACH INDIVIDUAL GATE WAS OF ONE PEARL, AND THE STREET OF THE CITY WAS PURE GOLD, LIKE TRANSPARENT GLASS. >

===================================

6   DIVINE DIMENSIONS

WELL WE HAVE NOW COME TO THE SIX CHAPTER OF MY BOOK, AND I REALLY HOPE IT HAS ALREADY BEEN A BLESSING TO YOU IN VARIOUS ASPECTS OF YOUR LIVES.

CONTRARY TO THE PRECEDING CHAPTERS, HERE IN THIS CHAPTER I AM GOING TO TELL YOU MAINLY OF AN EXPERIENCE THAT HAS HAPPENED TO ME PERHAPS ABOUT 13-15 YEARS AGO' IN MY MAIN CHURCH IN LONDON [KENSINGTON TEMPLE], I BELIEVE DURING A WEDNESDAY EVENING PRAYER MEETING. I AM SURE THAT YOU WILL AGREE THAT THIS IS AN ASTONISHING EXPERIENCE, AND I AM GLAD I AM WRITING TO BELIEVERS, THOUGH I STILL RECOGNISE THAT IT IS NOT A STORY EASY TO BELIEVE FOR ANYBODY, BECAUSE SADLY EVEN WITH THE ENLIGHTENING OF THE SCRIPTURES, OUR REDEMPTION AND THE DWELLING THE HOLY SPIRIT IN OUR HEARTS, OUR HUMAN AND SINFUL NATURE CAUSE MUCH DIFFICULTIES, SEPARATION AND IGNORANCE, WITHIN OURSELVES, BETWEEN US AND GOD AND HIS SCRIPTURES. FOR THIS PURPOSE TOO I AM INCLUDING IN THIS CHAPTER, I BELIEVE AN IMPORTANT AND INTERESTING THEOLOGICAL COMMENT AND REFLECTION ON THE FOLLOWING STORY, TO OPEN IT UP AND ANALYSE IT IN THE LIGHT OF THE SCRIPTURES AND OUR DAILY LIVES.AND TO STIR YOUR CURIOSITY EVEN LITTLE MORE, I WOULD LIKE TO ASK OURSELVES THIS FOLLOWING QUESTION: WHY IS GOD'S IMAGE REFERRED IN THE PLURAL THEN AS WELL AS TODAY IN GEN 2, AND CONSEQUENTLY SHOULD THIS PLURALITY APPLIED TO MAN'S TOO?

BUT LET US MOVE ON AND SEE FURTHER.

NOW I DO NOT REMEMBER NOW IF I WAS STILL AT THE
END OF MY BIBLE COLLEGE STUDIES [IBIOL], OR I HAD
JUST FINISHED IN 99; ANYHOW I HAD SINCE 97 AT THE
END OF MY EVENING CERTICATE IN CHRISTIAN STUDIES, A
STRONG DESIRE TO BE RELEASED IN THE FULL TIME
MINISTRY DOING THE WORK OF THE LORD. THUS I OFTEN
DWELLED IN THESE THOUGHTS, ALMOST TO THE POINT
OF FRUSTRATION MANY TIMES, AND HOWEVER DESPITE I
HAVE NOT GOT IT JET [12-JULY-11], THE LORD HAS
GRACIOUSLY ENABLED ME, AND STILL DOES, TO DO A LOT
OF WORK FOR HIM WHILE FOCUSING ON HIS KINGDOM
FIRST AND ON HIS CROSS, EQUIPPING ME WITH HIS
GRACE, PATIENCE AND CONFORT, AS WELL AS GIVING ME
THE POWER TO SHUN THE MINISTRY AS AN IDLE PER SE'.

UNFORTUNATELY IN MY EARLY YEARS I HAD NOT
STUDIED MUCH, ALSO FOR REASONS THAT I HAVE
MENTIONED ALREADY IN THE INTRODUCTION, AND I
BELIEVE THAT MAYBE FOR THIS LACK OF KNOWLEDGE
ALSO, THAT WHEN I HAD ASKED TO BE INVOLVED IN THE
MINISTRY IN OUR MAIN CHURCH [K.T., AT LEAST
INDIRECTLY], I FELT THAT I HAD BEEN UNFORTUNATELY
REJECTED. IF THAT WAS SO, NEVERMIND AND THEY WERE
PROBABLY RIGHT TO DO SO ANYHOW.

DESPITE ALL, I BELIEVE THAT IN THE FOLLONWING YEARS
OF BIBLE COLLEGE, THAT IS 98-99, THE LEADERS BEGAN

TO SEE THE GENUINITY AND POTENTIAL OF MY CALLING
IN CHRIST JESUS, AND SO I BELIVE THAT AT TIMES I FELT
THAT THEY PERHAPS WERE GIVING ME SIGNALS THAT
THEY WANTED TO TALK TO ME AND TO PROPOSE
SOMETHING TO ME IN THESE TERMS.

BUT IT NEVER HAPPENED SO FAR, CERTAINLY FOR MUCH
OF MY FAULT AS PERHAPS I WAS A BIT AFRAID, TOO
TIMID, OR EVEN MAYBE UPSET OR TOO RESERVED....OR
PERHAPS EVEN FOR SOME MISUNDERSTANDINGS WITH
THE LEADERS.

ANYHOW LET US NOW FIRSTLY LOOK AT GEN.1:26-27
WHICH TELLS THAT: < THEN GOD SAID, "LET US MAKE
MAN IN OUR IMAGE, ACCORDING TO OUR LIKENESS;..."
SO GOD CREATED MAN IN HIS OWN IMAGE; IN THE
IMAGE OF GOD HE CREATED HIM; MALE AND FEMALE HE
CREATED THEM. >

AS I MOVE ON, I KNOW THAT YOU ARE ALREADY WELL
AWARE THAT ESPECIALLY IN THOSE YEARS I WAS VERY
MUCH INVOLVED IN PRAYER, INTERCESSION, WORSHIP
AND EVANGELISTIC WORK TOWARDS PEOPLE OF ALL
NATIONS AND PERSONAL FRIENDS TOO. SO IT HAPPENED
THAT ON A WEDNESDAY EVENING, AS I WAS USED TO, I
WAS IN OUR MAIN CHURCH FOR THE PRAYER MEETING.
NORMALLY THIS SERVICE WOULD INCLUDE A TIME OF
WORSHIP, A GOOD TIME OF PRAYER AND INTERCESSION,

[A VERY IMPORTANT ELEMENT AS SOME WOULD SAY THAT HISTORY BELONGS TO THE INTERCERRORS AS SEEN IN DANIEL 9], AND LASTLY A SMALL SERMON, OCCASIONALLY SOME TIME FOR MINISTRY TOO.

IN THAT PARTICULAR EVENING, I THINK THE SECTION OF WORSHIP HAD ALREADY FINISHED, AND WE WERE NOW BEING TAKEN UP IN THE TIME OF INTERCESSION AIMING AT VARIOUS RELEVANT GOALS. JUST BEFORE THE LEADER WOULD DISCUSS IN ADVANCE SO THAT ALL, IN ALL FREEDOM AS THE EACH WAS LED IN HIS HEART, IN LOUD [AND I MEAN LOUD] PRAYERS AND SHOUTS WOULD JOIN IN TOGETHER. THIS FOLLOWING PARTICULAR I REMEMBER IT, AS IF IT WAS TODAY!

THIS IS WHAT I MEAN, AS WE WERE STANDING, IN A FEW SECONDS OF INTERVAL AS I WAS PRAYING WITH EVERYBODY ELSE, AS AT TIME I BELIEVED WE ALL DO, I ALSO INJECTED IN THE PRAYER BASKET OF MY MIND AND HEART A SPECIAL NEED OF MINE TOO.

WHAT WAS THIS SPECIAL NEED OF MINE? IT WAS ABOUT JUST WHAT I HAVE BEN WRITING, THAT IS I WAS TRYING TO UNDERSTAND WHY SOMEHOW INSIDE ME, THOUGH I DESIRED VERY MUCH TO BE IN THE FULL TIME MINISTRY, AT THE SAME TIME I SEEMED TO BE STRUGGLING WITH ACCEPTING THIS IDEA OF CHANGING MY LIFE IN SUCH A PROFOUND WAY, AND THUS I WAS ACTUALLY SOMEHOW AT LEAST PARTIALLY REJECTING IT MYSELF AND KEEPING

AWAY FROM CERTAIN LEADERS. I MUST CONFESS THAT PERHAPS THIS ATTITUDE OF MINE TRIGGERED ALSO SOME FUTURE DIRECT REJECTIONS BY SOME LEADERS TOWARDS MY VARIOUS REQUESTS TO BE MORE INVOLVED IN THE MINISTRY. ANYHOW THE LORD JESUS WAS TRULY THE REJECTED PER EXELLENCE, AND HE IS VERY MUCH QUALIFIED TO SYMPATHISE AND CONFORT US ALL.

AND SO IT WAS ABOUT THIS ISSUE THAT I STARTED TO PRAY ABOUT WITH ALL MY HEART JUST FOR MAYBE 5-10 SECONDS IN LOUD TOUNGES AND INTELLIGIBLE WORDS TOO; I NEEDED HELP, MORE UNDERSTANDING OF MYSELF WHICH WOULD DIRECT ME TOWARDS A SOLUTION!!!

SUDDENLY TO MY SHOCK, [AND IT MAY BE A SHOCK TO SOME OF YOU TOO AS YOU READ ON], AS SOON AS I STOPPED AND SHUT MY MOUTH AND KEPT SILENT, "SOMEONE ELSE" SPOKE TO, OR BETTER, IN ME, IN MY BOSOM. NOTE AGAIN THAT I WAS NOT DREAMING, OR DRUNK, OR SLEEPING, NOR WAS I IN DRUGS! THIS SPIRITUAL PERSON WITHIN ME SPOKE VERY CLEARLY IN ENGLISH SAYING, IN ANSWER TO MY PROBLEM AND ATTITUDE DILEMMA AS MENTIONED ABOVE, << BECAUSE I AM ALWAYS USED TO BE CURSED >>. DO NOTE AGAIN THAT HE DID NOT REFER TO ME AS "YOU ", BUT AS "I "!

AT THIS STAGE I AM TAKING FEW MOMENTS AGAIN FOR
THEOLOGICAL REFLECTION ON THE LINK BETWEEN GOD'S
AND MAN'S NATURE, IN PARTICULAR ON THE WORD "US
" USED BY GOD. WITH NO DISRESPECT, I BELIEVE THAT
I CANNOT AGREE WITH THOSE, STILL ON GEN. 1:26-27,
WHO THINK THIS IS A POINT OF GRAMMAR ALONE
WITHOUT A DIRECT BEARING ON THE MEANING, JUST
BECAUSE NO OTHER BEING HAS BEEN MENTIONED AND
AFTERWARDS ONLY THE SINGULAR IS USED, AND SO THIS
DOES NOT SPEAK OF NEITHER GOD'S NOR MAN' S
TRINITARIAN NATURE.

BUT WHAT DID THIS EXPERIENCE MEAN, WE MAY WANT
TO ASK? PERSONALLY I CAN SAY WITHOUT ANY DOUBT
AT ALL, THAT REALLY HE WAS NOT A DIFFERENT PERSON
SPEAKING WITHIN ME, BUT HE WAS ACTUALLY I MYSELF
IN THE PERSON OF MY PRE-EXISTENT OR UNBEGOTTEN
WORD/SON! AGAIN, IN CLEAR WORDS HE WAS THE
PERSON OF"MY WORD "!

WITHOUT DOUBT JOHN CHAPTER 1, ESPECIALLY VERSE 1
AND 18, WILL HELP YOU TO RECIEVE MORE
UNDERSTANDING ON THIS. HOWEVER FOR YOUR OWN
CURIOSITY, DO KNOW THAT ALREADY SINCE THE LAST
TWENTY YEARS AGO', I WAS REFLECTING ON THE
POSSIBILITY OF THE HUMAN INDIVIDUAL BEING
TRINITARIAN LIKE GOD, OBVIOUSLY NOT DIVINE BUT
HUMAN. AND I OFTEN DWELLED ON THIS TOPIC
ESPECIALLY IN TRYING TO UNDERSTAND MYSELF IN THE
CONTEXT OF MY DESIRES AND NEEDS TOWARDS THE
OTHER SEXUAL GENDER.

NOTE THAT ONE THING IS SPEAKING ABOUT ENERGIES AND ANOTHER IS SPEAKING ABOUT PERSONS IN RELATIONS!!!

PLEASE KEEP IN MIND THAT I KNOW CLEARLY THAT THIS WAS NOT THE VOICE OF GOD, NOR OF A DEMON EITHER, AS I KNOW HOW TO DISCERN THEM WELL, KNOWING WHAT THEY BOTH SOUND LIKE. INTERESTINGLY WE ALSO KNOW THAT THE SON OF GOD IS ALSO REFERED TO AS THE WISDOM OF GOD IN 1 COR. 1:18-2:31; [CF. ALSO PROV. 8].

AT THE SAME TIME THERE WAS WISDOM IN THIS VOICE WITHIN MY BOSOM!!!

IN FACT I AM SURE THAT IT IS THE CASE FOR MANY PEOPLE THAT WHEN FACING THE PROSPECT OF A NEW SITUATION IN THEIR LIVES THAT WOULD TAKE THEM TO AN HIGHER LEVEL OF LIFE STYLE, THEY WOULD CERTAINLY STRUGGLE WITH ALL KIND OF FEARS, FEELINGS OF DISCONFORTS AND SO ACTIVILY BRINGING TO THEMSELVES ALL KIND OF NEGATIVE QUESTIONS, DOUBTS WITH NEGATIVE POSSIBILITIES COMING TO THEIR MINDS IN ORDER TO PUT THEMSELVS OFF BY THEMSELVS, AND SO TO HINDER THEMSELVES FROM RECIEVE GOD'S BLESSING. IN FACT THESE HAVE BEEN SO USED TO THEIR LOW AND ALMOST CURSED LIFESTYLES, WHICH THEY NOW LIKE IT AND CHERISH IT WITHIN THEMSELVS, ALMOST SCARED TO LOOSE EVEN THE LITTLE

THAT THEY HAVE, WHILE STEPPING IN THE UNKNOWN. SO THEY REALLY ARE DIVIDED WITHIN THEMSELVES, IN WHAT THEY REALLY WANT TO DO, AND SO TAKING ANY DECISIONS BECOME HIGHLY PROBLEMATIC TO THEIR GREAT LOSS.

AND SO WHAT DOES IT MEAN GOD'S REFERENCE TO HIS BOSOM IN JOHN 1:18, AS FAR AS MAN'S IS CONCERN???

AND SO THIS WAS PARTIALLY MY CASE, AND I THINK THAT EVEN TODAY, I MAY BE DEALING WITH SOME FRAGMENTATIONS OF THIS STATE OF SPIRIT AND MIND, IF I CAN USE THESE WORDS, SINCE AS YOU HAVE PROBABLY UNDERSTOOD FROM THE INTRODUCTION, SOME EVENTS IN MY EARLY AGE HAD AFFECTED MY ATTITUDE TOWARDS LIFE IN A PARTICULAR AND DRAMMATIC WAY, THOUGH MAYBE I LEARNED A LOT FROM IT AND THROUGH GOD'S HELP HAVING OVERCOME, I CAN ALSO HELP OTHERS TO OVERCOME TOO. AND SO THANKS BE TO GOD FOR HIS TRANSFORMING POWER TODAY [MARK 5:21-43]. WELL HAVING SAID THIS THAT EVENING WENT ON AS USUAL AFTER THIS EXPERIENCE AND I CERTAINLY KEPT THE MATTER IN MIND, AS I STILL DO TODAY.

AT THIS POINT I WOULD LIKE TO SHARE WITH YOU WHAT FOLLOWS JUST BELOW, THAT IS: A THEOLOGICAL REFLECTION, COMMENT AND SMALL RESEARCH THAT I HAVE MADE ON THE HUMAN NATURE AS CREATED BY

OUR GOD IN HIS IMAGE AND LIKENESS. I BELIEVE THIS TO BE VERY IMPORTANT AND INTERESTING TOO, AND I HOPE IT WILL SEEM SO TO YOU TOO, BRINGING BLESSINGS TO YOUR LIVES IN A GENERAL AS WELL AS IN A PARTICULAR RELEVANT WAY, TO THE GLORY OF GOD.

NOW AS CHRISTIANS WE MUST ALL TRY SEE THE GREAT URGENCY FOR THE CHURCH TO DO ITS WORK IN THE WORLD AS ALWAYS AND TODAY MORE THAN EVER.

MY LITTLE CONTRIBUTION, I HOPE, WHICH I WOULD LIKE TO MAKE, IS AS FOLLOWS:

AS ALWAYS WE MUST FIND OUR RESOURCES IN THE GOSPEL/BIBLE, AND SO HERE MY FOCUS IS MORE ON HOW THE GOSPEL IS PREACHED BY THE CHURCH.

I BELIEVE BOTH THE BIBLE AND THE WORLD NEED TO PREACH AND HEAR A MORE COMPLETE, PRECISE AND RELEVANT GOSPEL AT LEAST FROM A CERTAIN, BUT VERY IMPORTANT ASPECT!

WHAT I MEAN IS THAT THE BIBLICAL GOSPEL OF THE KINDOM IS NOT JUST ONE OF SALVATION BUT ALSO OF CREATION [GEN 1-2; ETC...]; AND I THINK THE CHURCH LEAVES TOO MUCH OF A GAP OR GREY AREA BETWEEN THE TWO.

THIS IS WHERE WE NEED TO PAUSE BECAUSE, AS YOU KNOW TOO, ONE OF THE WORST OBSTACLE FROM RECIEVING THE GOSPEL IN THE WORLD TODAY, IS THE LACK OF UNDERSTANDING WELL THE TRINITARIAN NATURE OF THE GOD OF THE BIBLE, IN PARTICULAR ALSO IN RELATION TO OUR HUMAN NATURE!

AND THE SECOND WORST [IF NOT THE FIRST] OBSTACLE IS QUITE SIMILAR, THAT IS: NEITHER DOES THE CHURCH TEACH AND PREACH IT PROPERLY, NOR DO MOST PEOPLE UNDERSTAND THEMSELVES AS THEY BIBLICALLY AND REALLY ARE! IT IS JUST ONE BIG ISSUE REALLY!

JUST BECAUSE WE HAVE RECIEVED THE HOLY SPIRIT AND SALVATION, IT DOES NOT MEAN THAT WE VAVE A SOUND OR FAIRLY COMPLETE SPIRITUAL KNOWLEDGE OF OURSELVES!

AS IT IS KNOWN THE BIBLE, DOES NOT JUST REVEAL TO US GOD AND CREATION BUT ALSO MAN.

REMAINING IN THIS TOPIC:

* IT IS ON OUR LAST POINT, THE DOCTRINE OF MAN, THAT WE MUST SEE AGAIN OUR THEOLOGY. *

PLEASE FOLLOW ME FOR A LITTLE WHILE. I BELIEVE THAT WE COULD SEE THE WORDS "IMAGE AND LIKENESS ", AS MORE OR LESS MEANING THE SAME THING. MOREOVER WE CAN SEE EVEN FROM GEN. 9:6 AND JAMES 3:9.THAT THIS IMAGE/LIKENESS IS A PERMANENT ASPECT OF OUR CREATED NATURE, OR EVEN BETTER I WOULD SAY IT IS THE MOST IMPORTANT ASPECT OF OUR NATURE, AND SO HAS NOT BEEN LOST!

BUT LET US SEE TOGETHER JAMES 3:9: < WITH IT WE BLESS OUR GOD AND FATHER, AND WITH IT WE CURSE MEN, WHO HAVE BEEN MADE IN THE SIMILITUDE OF GOD. >

CERTAINLY IT HAS BEEN DISTORTED BY SIN, AS OUR VIRTUES AND ABILITIES.

BUT WHAT ABOUT UNDERSTANDING THE TRINITARIAN NATURE OF MAN AND GOD AS EVIDENCED AND LINKED BY THE LITTLE WORDS "US AND OUR"" IN GEN. 1:26?

I STRONGLY BELIEVE THAT WE NEED TO DISTINGUISH THE BIBLICAL MAN FROM OTHER IDEAS OF MAN!

I MUST SAY THAT AFTER HAVING MADE A WIDE THEOLOGICAL RESEARCH AMONG IMPORTANT AUTHORS, I COULD NOT SEE A PROPER ANALOGY/ EXPLANATION

FROM THE HUMAN PERSPECTIVE, THOUGH I HAVE APPRECIATED MANY USUFUL ELEMENTS!

AT THIS STAGE I WOULD LIKE TO ASK YOU TO FOLLOW ME JUST A LITTLE LONGER.

OBSERVE 2 VERY CRUCIAL POINTS:

1-- GEN 1:26 DEFINES THE ADAMIC NATURE AND LIKENESS IN GOD WITH THE PURAL "US AND OUR" OF ONE GOD! [NOTE THE SMALLNESS OF THESE WORDS AND SATAN'S SUCCESS IN WIPING THEM OUT FROM MOST PEOPLE].

IT IS INTERESTING AS THE TEXT DOES NOT MENTION IMAGES BUT "OUR IMAGE".

WHY?

BECAUSE THE BIBLE TELLS US THAT EACH PERSON OF THE TRINITY BEARS THE SAME AND UNCORRUPTED IMAGE [JOHN 10:30 WICH SAYS: < "I AND MY FATHER ARE ONE" >; 2 COR.4:4; JOHN 14:16, A COUNSELLOR OF THE SAME KIND, ...WHO THEN LOOKS THE SAME AS JESUS].

THIS IS QUITE RIGHTLY SO!

2--- GEN 3:5 IS ALSO VERY IMPORTANT.

NOTE AGAIN THE SMALL WORD "LIKE " HERE.

TILL RECENTLY I ALWAYS THOUGHT, FROM MY STUDIES
AND OTHERS' SERMONS [...TRUE TOO], THAT SATAN'S
SCHEME HAD ONLY TO DO WITH THE FACT THAT HE WAS
CAUSING EVE TO DOUBT GOD'S GOODWILL,
OVERSTRESSING THE STRICTNESS OF HIS COMMAND,
AND OFFERING SPIRITUAL ADVANTAGE, AND MAYBE
STIMULATING HER TO BECOME AN INDEPENDENT AND
SELF-SUFFICIENT CREAUTURE, AND SO
SEPARATING HUMANS FROM GOD.

HOWEVER I DESIRE TO ADD A VERY IMPORTANT ELEMENT
HERE, JUST UNDERSTOOD FEW DAYS AGO'.

I BELIEVE THAT SATAN'S MORTAL AND DESTRUCTIVE
ATTACK WAS ALSO AND ESPECIALLY, AIMED AT THE
HUMAN LINK TO GOD: HIS LIKENESS AND IMAGE IN
GOD < "FOR GOD KNOWS THAT IN THE DAY YOU EAT OF
IT YOUR EYES WILL BE OPENED, AND YOU WILL BE LIKE
GOD, KNOWING GOOD AND EVIL." > [GEN 3:5]!

PLEASE OBSERVE THESE TWO WORDS HERE: 'LIKE GOD'!?!
PERHAPS HE SOMEHOW TRIED TO RECREATE MAN, OR
MAN'S DEA OF HIS NATURE.

MAN'S IDEA OF HIMSELF WAS AND IS HERE MORE MADE
" LIKE " GOD AS IN TERMS OF KNOWLELDGE AND MORAL
INDEPENDENCE, THAT IS OF KNOWING GOOD AND EVIL!!!

***I FIND THIS A TERRIBLE SATANIC LIE WHICH
SOMEHOW GREATLY INFLUENCE OUR WORLD TODAY***

DRAWING NOW TOWARDS MY CONCLUSION, LOOKING
AT GEN 1:26, IN MY JUST MENTION FIRST POINT, MY
VIEW OF GOD'S IMAGE AND LIKENSS IN MAN IS AS
FOLLOWS:

***THOUGH HUMAN AND NOT DIVINE, ADAM WAS AND
IS A TRINITARIAN SPIRITUAL BEING, AS WELL AS, BUT NOT
JUST, A "SPIRIT-PSYCHO-BODY UNIT", AS WE MAY LEARN
IN OUR LIVES, SCHOOLS AND CHURCHES WITH ALL THE
QUALITIES AND ABILITIES THAT WE CAN THINK OF***

****THAT IS, AS FOR GOD:

1-THE SPIRITUAL MAN IS THREE PERSONS.

2- EACH PERSON IS FULLY SPIRITUAL MAN.

3- THERE IS ONE SPIRITUAL MAN.

******* THIS IS MAN'S IMAGE AND LIKENESS IN GOD IN
GEN 1:26-27 *******

TO THE SPIRITUAL AND BIBLICAL EYE THE SPIRITUAL MAN
IS EXPRESSESD AND MANIFESTED IN THREE PERSONS,
THOUGH USUALLY THIS IS NOT EVEN NOTICED, FELT OR
UNDERSTOOD BECAUSE OF THE CONSEQUENCE OF THE
FALL TO US! THIS INCLUDES ALSO THE CONSEQUENT FACT
THAT, THE LENGTH OF LIFE HAS BEEN MUCH SHORTENED,
WHILE THE ANCIENTS USED TO LIVE HUNDREDS OF
YEARS, NOW WE DO NOT HAVE EVEN ENOUGH TIME TO
REACH AN UNDERSTANDING OF OURSELVES, THAT WE
COULD HAVE REACHED, IF WE HAD LIVED FIVE OR SIX
HUNDREDS YEARS [CF. GEN. 5-6].

*** REFLECTING ALSO ON MY PAST STUDIES AND
KNOWLEDGE ABOUT GOD, WE SEE THAT ADAM MUST
BE "SOMEHOW" A LIVING BEING...AND LIKE A ROTATION,
[THOUGH I ADMIT I DO NOT FULLY UNDERSTAND THIS!]
OF THREE SPIRITUL PERSONS-IN-RELATION.

THAT IS:

1} AS FATHER [I COULD SAY THE VISIBLE AND SPIRITUAL
PERSON IN A WAY, THOUGH ALSO WHAT WE SEE WHEN
WE LOOK AT SOMEONE IS ALREADY: ONE IN
THREE: TRINITY; MOREOVER IN ALL THE HUMILITY OF MY
HUMAN STATE, I ADMIT THAT I DO NOT FIND IT EASY TO
GO INTO DEEPER AND MORE PRECISE DETAILS ON THIS
ISSUE, EXCEPT THAT I TRY TO TAKE PROTECTION

BY REMAINING WITHIN THE GUIDELINES OF THE
SCRIPTURES!].

2} THE PRE-EXISTENT PERSON OF THE HUMAN
WORD/SON IN THE BOSOM [CF. JOHN 1:1, 18].

3} AND THE PROCEEDING/GOING FORTH PERSON OF THE
HUMAN SPIRIT [CF. JOHN 14-16, WHO MEDIATES AND
REVEALS THE FATHER AND SON]. ***

NOW LET US FIRSTLY LOOK AT THIS GREAT VERSE OF
JOHN1:18: < NO ONE HAS SEEN GOD AT ANY TIME. THE
ONLY BEGOTTEN SON, WHO IS IN THE BOSOM OF THE
FATHER, HE HAS DECLARED HIM. > GOOD IS IT NOT? THE
TRUTH IS THAT OUR GOD IS THE ONLY WONDERFUL
COUNSELLOR AND REVEALER [ISA. 9].

SECONDLY AT THIS POINT, HERE IS JUST A BRIEF
ILLUSTRATION ON THIS LAST TRINITARIAN PERSON: OUR
PROCEEDING HUMAN SPIRIT. NOT THAT I THINK I HAVE
ANYTHING TO TEACH YOU, BUT I AM SURE THAT YOU
CAN AGREE WITH ME TO HAVE NOTICED THESE TWO
IMPORTANT FOLLOWING FACTORS, AND OTHERS TOO:

1- NOW WHEN WE ARE FORMING A QUEUE TO BUY A
COFFE AT A COFFESHOP; DO NOT WE AT TIMES FELL THE
SPIRITUAL PROMPTING OF THE PERSON BIHIND US
GIVING US 'SIGNS/FEELINGS' TO HURRY UP AND EVEN TO
GET LOST?

2-AT TIME WE DO LOOK INTENSILY AT AN ATTRACTIVE WOMAN WHO CAN BE WALKING EVEN ON THE PAVEMENT ACROSS THE ROAD; DO THEY NOT AT TIMES FEEL SOMETHING, AND THEN TURN AROUND TO SEE WHO IS LOOKING AT THEM?

*COULD IT BE BECAUSE OF OUR PROCEEDING SPIRIT, AS HE REVEALS OF WHAT IS OURS, AND THAT AT TIMES HIS WORK IS NOT THAT HOLY AS WE WOULD LIKE IT TO BE [JOHN 16:13-14]? IN FACT THE LORD JESUS IN THIS PASSAGE TELLS THAT: < "HOWEVER, WHEN HE, THE SPIRIT OF TRUTH, HAS COME, HE WILL GUIDE YOU INTO ALL TRUTH; FOR HE WILL NOT SPEAK ON HIS OWN AUTHORITY, BUT WHATEVER HE HEARS HE WILL SPEAK; AND HE WILL TELL YOU THINGS TO COME. HE WILL GLORIFY ME, FOR HE WILL TAKE OF WHAT IS MINE AND DECLARE IT TO YOU. >

GOOD FOOD FOR THOUGHT, DO YOU NOT THINK SO? *

TAKE GOOD NOTE MOREOVER OF WHAT HAPPENED TO ME IN THESE FOLLOWING TWO BRIEF ACCOUNTS, PERHAPS BOTH IN EARLY 2014 AND WITHIN A FEW WEEKS FROM EACH OTHER. 1] ONE MORNING AS I WAS IN THE HOUSE AND STANDING IN THE LANDING ON THE FIRST FLOOR LOOKING DOWN THE STAIRS AND ON THE GROUND FOOR FLAT, I SAW LIKE COMING OUT OF ME AND GOING DOWN THE STAIRS TO THE GROUND FLOOR, SOMETHING LIKE A SHADOW/SPIRIT/CHILD SHAPE ABOUT

90CM HIGH, AND TO MY SURPRISE/SHOCK SO! WE DO LIKE SPACIOUS PLACES, DO NOT WE?

2] PERHAPS A FEW WEEKS LATER AS I WAS WAITING FOR THE BUS, THE SAME EXPERIENCE HAPPENED TO ME, BUT THIS TIME THIS SHADOW/CHILD WENT TOWARDS THIS ATTRACTIVE WOMAN JUST ARRIVED TO THE BUS STOP, AND I SAW "HIM" AS RAISING HIS ARMS AS FOR PLAYING WITH HER OR TO BE LIFTED UP BY HER, AND SO TO MY SURPRISE AGAIN. [BY THE WAY IT MAY REMIND SOME OF YOU THE NEED TO SAY TO YOUR CHILDREN "COME BACK HERE".

PLEASE OBSERVE THE WORDS OF THE LAST PROPHET OF THE OLD TESTAMENT: MAL. 2:15 <...THEREFORE TAKE HEED TO YOUR SPIRIT...>

**** AS FOR GOD, IT IS ALSO AS FOR MAN, THOUGH HUMAN AND NOT DIVINE!

THESE ARE PARTAKERS OF THE SAME REALITY OF HUMAN BEING, FULLY BUT DISTINCT ONLY IN THAT EACH IS A DIFFERENT PERSON-IN-RELATION WITHIN THAT UNITARY SUBSTANCE/REALITY. ****

BECAUSE AS THE BIBLE SHOW US AS IN 2 COR. 13:14, AND THROUGHOUT IT:

***A]-THERE IS ONE GOD B]-GOD IS 3 PERSONS. 3]-EACH
PERSON IS FULLY GOD. ***

LET US BRIEFLY SEE SOME WORDS IN JOHN 1:1-4; 14: < IN
THE BIGINNING WAS THE WORD, ...AND THE WORD WAS
WITH GOD...ALL THINGS WERE MADE THROUGH HIM...IN
HIM WAS LIFE, AND THE LIFE WAS THE LIGHT OF
MEN...AND THE WORD BECAME FLESH AND DWELT
AMONG US, AND WE BEHELD HIS GLORY, THE GLORY AS
OF THE ONLY BEGOTTEN OF THE FATHER, FULL OF GRACE
AND TRUTH. >

I AM SURE YOU CAN SEE HERE IN THIS SMALL PASSAGE
SOME VITAL/LIFE-ESSENTIAL WORDS: GOD, MADE, LIFE,
LIGHT, MEN, FLESH, GLORY, FATHER, GRACE AND TRUTH!
IMPORTANT WORDS INDEED!

THUS JOHN TOLD THE GREEK AS WELL AS US, THAT GOD'S
DIVINE PRINCIPLE AND LIFE FORCE, THAT CREATED AND
SUSTAINS THE COSMOS, IS QUITE DIFFERENT FROM THE
GREEK IDEA 'IMPERSONAL' OF THE LOGOS! IN FACT THIS
HE IS A PERSON! HIM THEN BECAME INCARNATE 2,000
YEARS AGO' IN JESUS CHRIST OUR SAVIOUR; AND THIS
MAINLY THROUGH THE MIRACLE OF THE HOLY SPIRIT,
NOT THROUGH HUMANS WAYS AS THE CHILDREN OF
MEN GENERATE! *

PLEASE ALSO NOTE THE VARIOUS BIBLICAL REFERENCES
TO BOSOM; ZECH 12:1; JESUS AS THE LIFE AND TRUTH;
REV. 12:1-6; THE " I AM " OF BOTH TESTAMENTS AND THE
I AM OF THE PERSON OF THE HUMAN WORD IN OUR
BOSON RATHER THAN THE " I THINK OF DESCARTES ". IT
IS THIS TRUTHS AND CERTAINTIES, THAT CAN HELP US
TODAY, IN THE MIDST OF A GREAT HUMAN CRISES OF
CONFIDENCE AND CONSECRATION, TO BE BETTER
ESTABLISHED AND OPERATE IN AND FROM GOD'S
BIBLICAL AND TRUE KNOWLEDGE AND IDENTITY IN HIM
OUR MAKER [EX. 3:2; ISA 4:4; JOHN 8:12;58]. WE ARE
ALSO TO REFLECT ON GOD'S AFFERMATION TO US "THIS
IS MY SON" TAKEN CARE IN ETERNITY AS HIS WORD, AND
THE SO CALLED "THE ANGEL OF THE LORD" [EX. 3:2]; AND
THE ORIGIN OF THE FAMILY IN AND FROM GOD THE
FATHER [EPH. 3: 14-15]. SEE ALSO EPH 5: 22-33 IN PAUL'S
ANALOGY BETWEEN THE RELATIONSHIP OF HUSBAND
AND WIFE AND THE RELATIONSHIP BETWEEN GODS'S
SON AND THE CHURCH AS HIS BRIDE.

MOREOVER DO CAREFULLY NOTE THE ZEAL OF THE
ANGEL OF THE LORD FOR SEXUAL PURITY AND COVENANT
FAITHFULNESS, AS AN EXAMPLE AND AN
ENCOURAGEMENT TO US, AND IN COMPARISON TO OUR
BEHAVIOUR IN OUR TRINITARIAN DIMENSIONS, GREATLY
AFFECTED BY THE FALL IN IGNORANCE AND
BACKSLIDENESS. NO WANDER WHY I DO NOT REMEMBER

HEARING ANY PREACHER SPEAKING ON THIS PASSAGE OF EX. 4:24-25: < AND HE CAME TO PASS ON THE WAY, AT THE ENCAMPMENT, THAT THE LORD MET HIM AND SOUGHT TO KILL HIM. THEN ZIPPORAH TOOK A SHARP STONE AND CUT OFF THE FORESKIN OF HER SON AND CAST IT AT MOSES'S FEET, AND SAID, "SURELY YOU ARE A HUSBAND OF BLOOD TO ME!" > {PLEASE SEE 3:2 ALSO <...THE ANGEL OF THE LORD...>}.

I SAY THAT WAS A VERY HARD CHASSENING INDEED, AND WITHOUT ANESTHETIC!

NOW I BELIEVE THAT IN THE FALL SATAN TRIED TO REDUCE MEN ALMOST TO EMPTY MASKS/PERSONS.

I WANT TO COMMENT HERE, THAT THE ABOVE IS QUITE RIGHT: NO SON=NO LIFE=DEATH!

MOST PEOPLE ON EARTH TODAY ARE IN FACT UNAWARE OF THEIR TRINITARIAN SPIRITUAL SUBSTANCE/SPIRIT /INHERITANCE; AND LIKE EMPTY MASKS, SACRIFICE THEIR BODIES AND SPIRITS TO HADES IN SEXUAL IMMORALITY, ETC...

WITH ALL KIND OF ALTERNATIVE THEY TRY TO FILL THEIR SENSE OF INADEQUACY AND EMPTINESS. THE CONSEQUENCES ARE SPIRITUAL, MENTAL, PHYSICAL, ECONOMICAL OF THE HIGHEST COST...HUMANITY IS IN A TERRIBLE STATE...THE URGENCY TO DELIVER GOD'S

MESSAGE WORLD WIDE IS MUCH HIGHER THAN WHAT
WE CAN THINK OF!

NOW OUT OF INTEREST A FEW WEEKS AGO' ON THE 5TH
OF MAY I PARTICIPATED IN A CONFERENCE IN A CHURCH
VENUE HERE IN LONDON [EMMANUEL CENTRE, NEAR
WESTMINSTER ABBEY], LEAD BY THE ANGLICAN
MAINSTREAM WHICH IS A COMMUNITY WITHIN THE
ANGLICAN CHURCH COMMITTED TO PROMOTING
BIBLICAL TRUTHS. THE MAIN TOPIC OF THIS ASSEMBLY
WAS SEXUAL EDUCATION AND RELATIONSHIP IN OUR
SCHOOLS, AND ONE OF THE MAIN SPEAKERS WAS DR.
MIRIAM GROSSMAN FROM CALIFORNIA; SHE IS A
PHYSICIAN WITH TRAINING IN PAEDRIATICS AS WELL AS
PSYCHIATRY. WELL IT WAS VERY INFORMATIVE WITHOUT
DOUBT. BY THE WAY AT THE END OF THE CONFERENCE I
WAS ABLE TO SAY HELLO TO HER, AND BRIEFLY
PRESENTED TO HER THE CORE OF MY VIEW WHICH I AM
ALSO PRESENTING TO YOU HERE, AND SHE PLEASANTLY
AND RESPECTFULLY LISTENED, PERHAPS SHOWING SIGNS
OF SURPRISE THOUGH WITHOUT MAKING
ANY COMMENTS, BEING ALSO RATHER BUSY.

ANYHOW HERE I LEARNED THAT IT HAS BEEN
PROVED MEDICALLY THAT BEFORE A WOMAN KNOWS
THAT SHE IS PREAGNANT, THE BRAIN OF THE FOETUS IS
ALREADY MALE OR FEMALE! MOREOVER CROMOSONS

ARE DIFFERENT FOR EACH GENDER! A NOTION IN
AGREEMENT WITH THE SCRIPTURES AND VERY MUCH
CONTRARY TO THE SEEMINGLY RISING IDEA IN SOCIETY
THAT GENDER IS ONLY SOCIALLY CONSTRUCTED! ALSO I
LEARNED THAT IN TEENAGERS THE PART OF THE BRAIN
RESPONSABLE FOR MAKING DECISIONS [WISE
HOPEFULLY], IS ONLY COMPLETELY FORMED IN THE
MIDDLE TWENTIES; AN INFORMATION THAT SUGGESTS A
WORD OF ALARM, AND PRUDENCE AT LEAST AGAINST
THE FREQUENT CASES OF TEENAGERS PREGNANCIES IN
OUR SOCIETY WICH OFTEN END IN PAINFUL AND
DESTRUCTIVE ABORTIONS.

MUCH WAS ALSO SAID ABOUT CONSEQUENT SEXUAL
DEASESES AND THE FACT THAT CONDOMS REALLY OFFER
ONLY PARTIAL PROTECTION AGAINST THESE. TO MY
SHOCK I ALSO LEARNED THAT, IF I HAVE UNDERSTOOD
CORRECTLY, SOME OF THE TEACHINGS IN OUR SCHOOLS
ABOUT SEXUAL EDUCATION HAS BEEN INSPIRED OR
INTRODUCED BY AN AMERICAN SCHOLAR SEEN BY SOME
AS A DISTURBED INDIVIDUAL. THIS ALSO WANTED TO
PROMOTE CHILDREN SEXUALITY IN THE EDUCATIONAL
FIELD. I AM SURE THAT SOME OF YOU WHO ARE READING
THIS ARE MORE AWARE OF THE DETAILS REGARDING
WHAT I HAVE JUST MENTIONED ABOVE.

VERY BRIEFLY, TOUGH I RECOGNISE THAT I AM NOT
STRICTLY SPEAKING AN EXPERT IN THE MATTER OF
SEXUAL EDUCATION TO CHILDREN, I WOULD LIKE TO

REFLECT AND SAY THAT THE SCRIPTURES CERTAINLY ENCOURAGE GENERAL EDUCATION AGAINST IGNORANCE, BUT IT SHOULD BE DONE FROM THE BIBLICAL EXAMPLE, FOCUSING ON THE BETTER QUALITIES AND VALUES OF THE KINDOM OF GOD SUCH AS LOVE, AND THE SO CALLED FRUITS OF THE HOLY SPIRIT!

MOREOVER CHILDREN SHOULD HAVE THEIR INNOCENCE RESPECTED AND PROTECTED AND LIKE JESUS AND JOHN THE BAPTIST, SHOULD BE ALLOWED TO GROW IN SPIRIT, STATURE, WISDOM AND IN FAVOR WITH GOD AND MAN; AND NOT BEING ENCOURAGED TO BE TEMPTED AND FRUSTATED BY THE FLESHLY DESIRES; EITHER TO BE USED AS SEXUAL PRODUCTS FOR CONSUMPTION [LUKE 1:68; 2:52]! DO OBSERVE LUKE 2:52 < AND JESUS INCREASED IN WISDOM AND STATURE, AND IN FAVOUR WITH GOD AND MEN. >

PLEASE DO NOTE THAT TO GROW IN FAVOR WITH GOD AND MAN IS DIRECTLY THE OPPOSITE AS RECIEVING DESASES AND ALL KIND OF PROBLEMS AND CURSES FROM GOD, THE DEVIL AND MAN!

MOREOVER I WOULD ALSO ADD THAT NO DOUBT MANY ARE THE REASONS FOR SEXUAL PROBLEMS AND THEIR CONSEQUENCES, AS EACH PERSON FACES HIS/HER OWN PARTICULAR CONTEXT.

HOWEVER I WOULD LIKE TO SUGGEST THAT USUALLY IT ALL DERIVES FROM A PROBLEM OF PARENTING. WHAT I MEAN IS THAT GOD HIMSELF GAVE THE BEST EXAMPLE OF GOOD AND SOUND PARENTING IN ETERNITY AND ALL HOLINESS, AND WHEN HE DECIDED TO GENERATE HIS SON WAS NOT ASHAMED TO SAY BASICALLY THAT HERE HE WAS, THIS MY SON, LOOK AND LISTEN TO HIM!!! AND WHAT ABOUT US, ARE WE PROUD OF OUR PRE-EXISTENT "OURSELVES/SONS AND DAUGHTERS", THE PERSONS OF OUR 'WORDS' AS IN JOHN1:1-2, THAT IS NOT AS THE ANGEL OF THE LORD, BUT IN OUR HUMAN CASE: THE 'INVISIBLE' ANGELS OF MEN; [GEN. 16:10].

*** THE SO CALLED "INNER MAN", SPOKEN OF BY THE APOSTLE PAUL IN 2 COR. 4:16 AND EPH. 3:16 CANNOT BE IGNORED! *** [IF IT MAY BE TAKEN IN THIS CONTEXT].

SO THEN GOOD AND SOUND PARENTING STARTS FIRST WITH EVERY INDIVIDUAL IN HIS TRINITARIAN SPIRITUAL NATURE, MUCH BEFORE CONSIDERING MARRIAGE, THAT IS IN OUR BOSOM!!!

NOW ROUGHFULLY THE BIBLE SHOULD HAVE ONLY BEEN COMPOSED OF GEN. 1 AND 2! THE REST IS MOSTLY AN EXPLANATION OF IT, A FALL FROM IT, AND A RESTORATION TO IT.

JESUS DID NOT JUST COME TO REVEAL GOD, BUT ALSO MAN!

THE DEVIL COULD NOT SUCCEED TO DELETE THE SON AS BEING GOD, BECAUSE HE RESURRECTED; BUT HE IS CERTAINLY SUCCEEDING IN ROBBING MAN IN HIS AWARENESS AND UNDERSTANDING, OF HIS 2 SPIRITUAL PERSONS: HIS WORD AND HIS PROCEEDING FORTH SPIRIT.

AS FOR ME, PLEASE TAKE NOTE:

GOD GAVE HIS ONLY WORD SO THAT MAN COULD ALSO REFIND HIS! [JOHN1:1; MATTH 17:5]

PLEASE OBSERVE THAT THE DUTY OF THE CHURCH TODAY IS TO EQUIP AND RESTORE MAN WITH GOD'S FULNESS OF HIS IMAGE AND LIKENESS THROUGH THE HOLY SPIRIT AND THE BIBLICAL KNOWLEDGE OF HIS GOSPEL OF CREATION AND REDEMPTION, AND SO ALSO SPEED UP THE COMING OF THE LORD JESUS [MUCH MORE IMPORTANT THAN GETTING MANY DEGREES IN DISCEPLESHIP].

WE NEED TO DO THIS IN ALL THE WAYS WE CAN; AND THROUGH AL KINDS OF TOOLS OF COMMUNICATIONS WE MUST BOMBARD THE LIES OF SATAN WITH THE TRUTH OF

THE GOSPEL, AVOIDING ALSO RISKING OVERSTRESSING ANY TOOL OR STRATEGY!

AS SOME OF YOU MAY KNOW, IT TOOK LONG TIME FOR ITALY TO REACH THIS NATIONAL UNITY [1861], AS IT IS THIS YEAR CELEBRATING ITS 150 ANNIVERSARY, SO ALSO, MAN MUST UNDERSTAND AND REFIND HIS GOD'S GIVEN AND INTENDED SPIRITUAL UNITY AND NATURE AND COMPLETENESS WITHIN HIMSELF AND GOD.

MOREOVER OBSERVE THE IMPORTANCE/URGENCY OF THE FATHER/SON CALL FOR HARMONIOUS RELATIONSHIP AT THE HEART OF BIBLE, POINTING US AGAIN TO AN HARMONIOUS RELATIONSHIP WITHIN THE GODHEAD AND MANHEAD, AS WELL AS THE EXTERNAL RELATIONSHIP BETWEEN PARENTS AND CHILDREN [EZEK. 16:20; MAL.2:15-16; 4:6; LUKE 1:17; JOHN 14:17;16]!!!

THIS IS OF PRIMARY IMPORTANCE! IT ALL STARTS FROM HERE FIRST!

*** OF COUSE, SINCE GOD THE TRINITY ACTS SINGULARLY, SO DOES ALSO MAN THE TRINITY [CONSIDERING THE PRE-INCARNATE STATE OF HIS WORD TOO]; ALL THIS AVOIDING OVERSTRESSING, OR GOING CRAZY, OR TOO DEEP, OR IN UN UNBIBLICALLY DIRECTED WAY, ABOUT THESE SPIRITUAL DETAILS AND DIMENSIONS IN OUR MINDS AND ACTIONS! ***

IF WE CANNOT EVEN CONTROL OUR SPIRIT, WHERE IS OUR HOPE THEN?

AGAINST DIVORCE AND UNFAITHFUL BEHAVIOUR THE PROPHETS STILL REPEATEDLY CRY IN OUR SOCIETY << ...HE SEEKS GODLY OFFSPRING. THEREFORE TAKE HEED TO YOUR SPIRIT THAT YOU DO NOT DEAL TREACHEROUSLY WITH THE WIFE OF YOUR YOUTH... >> [MAL. 2:15-16].

IN FACT PROV. 16:32 TELLS THAT "HE WHO HE SLOW TO ANGER IS BETTER THAN THE MIGHTY, AND HE WHO RULES HIS SPIRIT, THAN HE WHO CAPTURES A CITY."

SO THEN IF WE ALSO DISTINGUISH THE BIBLICAL MAN IN THIS WAY, FROM ANY OTHER IDEAS OF MAN, WE SHALL BOTH UNDERMINE MANY FALSE BELIEFS THAT ARE ATTACKING OUR WORLD.

IN FACT OUR PRAYER IS TO SEE ALL PEOPLE IN HEAVEN; THAT NONE SHOULD PERISH [2PETER 3:9]; AND THAT ALSO MUSLIMS MAY DISCERN AND UNDERSTAND THAT NOT ONLY IS GOD TRINITARIAN: THAT HIS NAME IS TRINITY! BUT THAT ALSO THE NAME OF MAN IS TRINITY; BECAUSE BOTH GOD AND MAN REFLECT ONE ANOTHER'S TRINITARIAN NATURE!

WITHOUT THIS DIVINE/HUMAN DIMENSION THERE COULD NOT BE ANY MULTIPLICATION ON EARTH!

MOREOVER, AGAIN PRAYING THAT IT WILL BE SOON SO, I HAVE NO DOUBT THAT IF WE IN SOCIETY WOULD PROMOTE THE EDUCATION OF THESE TRUTHS IN OUR COLLEGES AND UNIVERSITIES, SOCIAL HURTS AND PROBLEMS, SUCH AS THE CASE OF HAVING HERE IN UK PERHAPS ABOUT 200,000 ABORTIONS PER YEAR AND OTHER ISSUES AS MENTIONED ABOVE, WOULD DIMINUISH FOR THE WELL BEING OF ALL, TO THE GLORY OF GOD, AMEN! THIS WOULD BE SO AS WELL AS FACILITATING THE UNDERSTANDING AND RECEPTION OF THE GOSPEL, IN THE HOPE, WITH GOD'S GRACE, OF MORE GENUINE CONVERSIONS AND MORE CULTURES AND COMMUNITIES IMPACTED AND TRANSFORMED BY THE BIBLICAL SCRIPTURES/GOSPEL WITH A NEW CONFIDENCE!

BASICALLY, I WOULD LIKE TO NOTE THAT, CONTRARY TO WHAT WE SOMETIMES DO TO OTHERS AND WITHIN TO OURSELVES WITH NEGATIVE THOUGHTS, AS EVEN NEGATIVE TOUGHTS ARE LIKE INNER CURSES, GOD'S TRINITARIAN PERSONS-IN-RELATION HONOUR AND PRAISE ONE ANOTHER AS IN MATTH. 3:17: < AND SUDDENLY A VOICE CAME FROM HEAVEN, SAYING, "THIS IS MY BELOVED SON, IN WHOM I AM WELL PLEASED." > AND SEE ALSO JOHN 5:19; 15:26!

BECAUSE TO THE GLORY AND FROM THE GLORY OF GOD, THE LEAST WE CAN SAY IS THAT WE CANNOT, DESPITE THE DEVIL'S SCHEMES, SEPARATE GOD'S TRINITARIAN IMAGE AND LIKENESS FROM OUR HUMAN TRINITARIAN IMAGE AND LIKENESS IN HIM. ON THE CONTRARY THESE BOTH REFLECT AND EXPRESS THEIR UNITY AND TRUTH: MAN IS NOT ANOTHER GOD, BUT DESPITE MANY OF HIS BAD INTENTIONS, HE IS AND CAN ONLY BE THE REPRESENTATIVE OF THE ONLY TRUE AND REAL GOD: THAT IS YAHWEH OF THE BIBLE! [EX 3; JOHN 10:30; 14:9-11; COL 1:15; HEBR. 1:3]. BUT SEE THE LORD JESUS IN JOHN 10:35-36: < "IF HE CALLED THEM GODS, TO WHOM THE WORD OF GOD CAME (AND THE SCRIPTURE CANNOT BE BROKEN), "DO YOU SAY OF HIM WHOM THE FATHER SANCTIFIED AND SENT INTO THE WORLD, 'YOU ARE BLASPHEMING,' BECAUSE I SAID, 'I AM THE SON OF GOD'? >

YES, JESUS IS THE SON OF GOD, AMEN!

THAT IS WHY HE IS ALSO THE SON OF MAN; AND SO MAN IS GOD'S REPRESENTATIVE ON EARTH, BEING MADE IN HIS OWN IMAGE AND LIKENESS, TO THE GLORY OF THE FATHER, AS IT WAS MEANT TO BE, AMEN [GEN. 1:26-27]!

================================

7   KINGDOM
REVELATIONS

WELL WITH GOD'S GRACE WE HAVE NOW ARRIVED TO OUR LAST CHAPTHER OF THIS BOOK. HERE I AM ABOUT TO TELL YOU OF OTHER FOUR LITTLE STORIES THAT HAVE HAPPENED TO ME DURING THESE LAST YEARS. I KNOW THAT I WILL NOT DISAPPOINT YOU, BUT I ALSO FEEL THAT I MAY PERHAPS TRIGGER IN YOU SOME KIND OF PERPLEXITY AND MAYBE EVEN, I HOPE, SOME KIND OF GODLY JELOUSY. WHATEVER, I SINCERELY WISH THAT YOU MAY BE ENCOURAGED, BUILD UP AND BLESSED IN YOUR READING OF THIS WITH THE PURPOSE ALSO IN BRINGING MORE GLORY TO THE KINGDOM OF OUR LORD AND SAVIOR JESUS, THE ANOINTED ONE.

NOW PLEASE DO PAY A PARTICULAR ATTENTION ON THE RIVER OF WATER OF LIFE IN REV. 22:1-2 FOR NOW, "AND HE SHOWED ME A PURE RIVER OF WATER OF LIFE, CLEAR AS CRYSTAL, PROCEEDING FROM THE THRONE OF GOD AND OF THE LAMB. IN THE MIDLLE OF ITS STREET, AND ON EITHER SIDE OF THE RIVER, WAS THE TREE OF LIFE, WHICH IT BORE TWELVE FRUITS, EACH TREE YEALDING ITS FRUIT EVERY MONTH. THE LEAVES OF THE TREE WERE FOR THE HEALINGS OF THE NATIONS."

HOWEVER I SHALL BE FOCUSING MAINLY ON THE WELL OF SALVATION SPOKEN OF IN JOHN 4!

NOW I AM SURE THAT YOU KNOW THAT MANY SCRIPTURES SEE AS WATER THE WISDOM OF THE LAW

AND SOMETIMES AS ALSO THE HOLY SPIRIT; ISA. 12:3; 55; 44:3; 49:1; PS. 36.

IT IS IN THIS CONTEXT THAT NOW THE FIRST STORY I AM ABOUT TO TALK TO YOU ABOUT IS SET; THIS HAPPENED TO ME PERHAPS IN 1995, POSSIBLY WHEN I HAD JUST BEGAN TO ATTEND THE EVENING CERTIFICATE IN CHRISTIAN MINISTRY IN OUR BIBLE COLLEGE. AGAIN IF THIS EXPERIENCE HAD NOT BEEN SUPPORTED BY THE SCRIPTURES, I WOULD HAVE BEEN VERY RELUCTANT TO WRITE IT. IT IS A FANTASTIC OR BETTER, A WONDERFUL EXPERIENCE FROM THE WONDERFUL SAVIOUR AND COUNSELLOR, AND THE ADDITIONAL MARVELLOUS FACT ABOUT IT, IT IS THAT I STILL EXPERIENCE IT TODAY ANYTIME I WANT TOO THANKS TO HIS GRACE; IT WAS NOT A ONE OFF EXPERIENCE!

BUT LET US NOW LOOK AT ISA. 44:3 TOGETHER, "FOR I WILL POUR WATER ON HIM WHO IS THIRSTY, AND FLOODS ON THE DRY GROUNDS; I WILL POUR MY SPIRIT ON YOUR DESCENDENTS, AND MY BLESSING ON YOUR OFFSPRING;"

AGAIN IN THAT TIME I WAS INVOLVED IN MUCH PRAYER AND INTERCESSION WITH MY CHURCH, TOWARDS VARIOUS TOPICS INCLUDING PRAYING FOR PEOPLE THAT I KNEW. PLEASE NOTE AGAIN THAT WHEN WE DO THINGS OR PRAY FOR OTHER PEOPLE WE ALSO GET BLESSED [CF.

JOHN 13:1-17]. I REMEMBER ONCE IN THE SATELLITE
CHURCH, THAT I WAS PRAYING FOR THE HEALING OF
SOMEONE'S EYES, AND TO MY SURPRISE, IN THE EVENING
IN THE MAIN CHURCH, I COULD READ THE WORDS IN THE
SCREEN BETTER THAN I USED TO; THOUGH I DO NOT
REMEMBER THE RESULT OF MY PRAYERS TOWARDS THAT
PERSON WHOM I WAS PRAYING FOR, I HAD BEEN HEALED
MYSELF, THANKS BE TO GOD. NOW, BACK TO THE
WEDNESDAY EVENING PRAYER MEETING, AS USUALLY I
USED TO SIT UPSTAIRS, AS I FELT AT THAT TIME TO BE
MORE INTIMATE WITH THE LORD. I DO NOT WANT TO
SEEM TO YOU TOO REPETITIVE, BUT AS YOU KNOW IN
THAT TIME I WAS VERY ZELOUS AND ACTIVE IN
EVANVELISM TOO, TAKING ADVANTAGE OF THE MANY
OPPORTUNITIES HERE IN LONDON.

I BELIEVE THAT WE COULD TAKE FOR "REAL WATER", THE
SPIRIT AND THE WORDS COMMUNICATED BY JESUS (ACTS
2:38; JOHN 7:39; HEBR. 6:4).

WELL THAT EVENING IN THE CHURCH, I REMEMBER THAT
I WAS INTERCEEDING A LOT FOR MY TWO WOMEN
FRIENDS, ONE ITALIAN AND ONE IRANIAN: FOR THEM TO
BE SAVED AND TO BE COMMITTED TO THE LORD. THEY
WERE BOTH LIVING SINFUL LIVES FAR AWAY FROM A
GODLY MODEL, AND IN MY CARING ZEAL, I WAS
PLEADING WITH THE LORD FOR A CHANGE IN THEIR
LIVES; MOREOVER I WAS ALSO IN FIRE BOTH FOR THE
LORD, AS WELL AS AGAINST THE DEVIL WHO HAD DONE

DAMAGE IN THE PAST TO BOTH ME AND MY FAMILY! I
KNOW SADLY THAT YOU TOO BEAR YOUR SCARS.

TO GIVE YOU JUST A SMALL EXAMPLE OF THIS, THE ONLY
BROTHER OF MY MOTHER, THOUGH HE WAS ONE OF THE
BEST STUDENTS IN HIS SCHOOL WHERE HE WAS
STUDYING LAW, SUDDENLY THINGS BEGAN TO GO
WRONG FOR HIM AND HE SPENT THE REST OF HIS LIFE IN
A PSYCHIATRIC HOSPITAL, THANK GOD WITH A LARGE
OPEN AIR SPACE, AND THE LAST FEW YEARS WITH OTHER
PATIENTS IN A KIND OF " FAMILY HOUSE ", BEING
DRUGGED ALL HIS LIFE; I BELIEVE ALSO HAVING HAD TO
SUBMIT A FEW TIMES TO [PERHAPS BARBARIC] ELECTRIC
CONVULSIONS, AND A CERTAINLY FAR FROM AN
HONORABLE LIFESTYLE. HE DYED A FEW YEARS AGO', AND
I AM SURE THAT SOON I SHALL MEET HIM IN PARADISE IN
MUCH BETTER CIRCUMSTANCES.

ANYHOW NOTE AGAIN THAT THIS WAS THE
SURROUNDING CONTEXT AND ATTITUDE OF MINE AT
THAT TIME WHEN I HAD THIS EXPERIENCE. REALLY WHAT
HE AND MANY OTHERS NEEDED WAS TO MEET JESUS AT
THE WELL, AS THE SAMARITAN WOMAN DID, HEARING
THE REAL GOSPEL!!!

DURING THE SEVICE, AFTER THE TIME OF WORSHIP
WHICH LASTED ABOUT 30-40 MINUTES, NORMALLY THE
PASTOR MUST HAVE BEEN PRESENTING THE VARIOUS
TOPICS FOR INTERCESSION; THEN OFTEN WE USED TO

PRAY FOR ONE TOPIC, AS USUALLY QUITE LOUD WITH THE POWER AND AUTHORITY THAT WE ENJOY IN CHRIST AND IN A SPIRIT OF FREEDOM AS EACH FELT LEAD TO SPEAK IN THEIR OWN WORDS, AND OF COURSE ALL TOGETHER.

THEN AFTER PRAYING ABOUT ONE TOPIC, THE PASTOR WOULD EXPAND THE NEXT CONTEXT AND TOPIC OF PRAYER AND SO AGAIN ALL THE ASSEMBLY WOULD LIFT UP THEIR VOICE IN PRAYER AGAIN. NOW IN THE MIDDLE OF THIS TIME AND ATMOSPHERE OF PRAYER, THAT I LIKE MANY OTHERS I GUESS WOULD DO, I WOULD SQUEEZE IN PERSONAL PRAYERS FOR ME AND MY FRIENDS, KNOWING ALSO THAT MY VOICE WOULD HAVE BEEN COVERED BY EVERYBODY ELSE'S VOICE.

NOW AS I WAS IN THE SERVICE, SUDDENLY SOMETHING EXTRAORDINARY AND MARVELLOUS HAPPENED TO ME. IT WAS LIKE AS THE HOLY SPIRIT HAD BROUGHT ME IN A NEW DIMENSION, ENABLING ME TO EXPERIENCE A NEW WAY OF 'LIVING', OR BETTER, "" A NEW AND ADDITIONAL WAY OF BREATHING "" !!!

BACK TO MY STORY AGAIN, YES, TO MY SHOCK, I FOUND MYSELF AS BEING ENABLED TO BREATH FROM WITHIN ME, TO DRAW AND DRINK REFRESHING PURE AIR FROM WITHIN MYSELF!!! IT WAS JUST AS ASTONISHING AS WONDERFUL!!!

THUS I THINK BOTH I AND THIS SAMARITAN WOMAN
WERE ACTUALLY IN THE RIGHT TIME, IN THE PLACE
CHOSEN BY GOD TO BE BLESSED!!!

BY THE WAY AT THAT TIME THE SERVICE USED TO BE FULL
BOTH IN THE GROUND FLOOR AS WELL AS UPSTAIRS;
ALSO THERE WAS NO AIR CONDITIONING IN THOSE
YEARS. PLEASE DO NOTE THAT THOUGH I HAD BEEN
FILLED WITH THE HOLY SPIRIT AT THE END OF 93, I NEVER
HAD EXPERIENCED ANYTHING OF THE SORT, NEITHER DID
I DREAM OF SUCH A THING TO BE AVAILABLE AND
POSSIBLE FOR THE INDIVIDUAL. BUT WE KNOW
HOWEVER THAT THE SCRIPTURES ARE FILLED WITH
TREASURES, SOME OF WHICH PERHAPS HAVE NOT BEEN
DISCOVERED JET.

I AM SURE THAT YOU WILL UNDERSTAND ME, PUTTING
YOURSELF IN MY SHOES, THAT THAT PARTICULAR
EVENING I DRUNK A LOT OF IT, AND EVEN FOR THE NEXT
FEW MONTHS. NOTE THAT THIS EXPERIENCE ONLY
REQUIRES ME TO MAKE THE GENTLE EFFORT TO DRAW IT,
OR SUCK IT FROM WITHIN ME, AND TO BE FAIRLY PURE
IN MY HEART TOWARDS THE LORD JESUS.

WE CANNOT BUT SEE THIS WONDERFUL VERSE IN JOHN
4:10, " JESUS ANSWERED AND SAID TO HER, "IF YOU
KNEW THE GIFT OF GOD, AND WHO IT IS WHO SAYS TO
YOU, 'GIVE ME A DRINK,' YOU WOULD HAVE ASKED HIM,
AND HE WOULD HAVE GIVEN YOU LIVING WATER."

YES, IT IS ABOUT JESUS ALWAYS, AS HE IS BOTH OUR SAVIOUR AND CREATOR.

I AM SURE THAT BOTH YOU AND I WOULD LIKE TO SAY AMEN TO THIS!

NOW IN MY CASE IT IS ALMOST LIKE AS HAVING AN INBUILT AND NOW UNBLOCKED CHANNEL WITHIN ME, THE MORE PURE I AM TOWARDS THE LORD, THE MORE CLEAR THE CHANNEL IS AND THE MORE I CAN DRINK OF IT, AND VICE VERSA. THUS I EXPERIENCE THIS ANY TIME I WANT TO AND DURING ALL THESE YEARS FROM 95 TILL DEC. IN 2011, I HAVE NEVER BEEN UNABLE TO ENJOY IT! I DO IT IN MY FREE WILL CONSTANTLY, SOMETIMES ONCE OR A FEW TIMES A DAY, SOMETIMES NOT FOR A FEW DAYS, THOUGH I AM ALWAYS CONSCIOUS OF IT. I ENJOY IT BOTH IN SUMMER AS IN WINTER, AND IT IS MY BEST REFRESHING DRINK, FREE OF CHARGE TOO, AND IT NEVER RUNS OUT!!! IT IS A REFILLING, REFRESHING AND SATISFYING "HOBBY", IF I MAY BE ALLOWED TO SPEAK LIKE THIS...

BUT VERY HUMBLY I KNOW THAT THIS WELL OF SALVATION WAS MADE AVAILABLE FOR US AT THE PRICE OF THE CROSS OF OUR SAVIOUR [JOHN 3:16].

THE ONLY THING IS THAT I CANNOT "OVER DO IT ", AS IF I KEPT DRAWING AND DRAWING, IT WOULD BECOME OVERPOWERING AND I WOULD NOT BE ABLE TO CONTAIN IT, AND PROBABLY FALL ON THE FLOOR. IN

TRUTH AND REALITY, WITHOUT DOUBT I KNOW THAT THE GREATEST BLESSING IS TO BE BORN AGAIN [REGENERATED BY THE HOLY SPIRIT], AND BEING FILLED WITH THE HOLY SPIRIT; HOWEVER I BELIEVE THAT THIS IS ALSO AN ADDITIONAL BLESSING AVAILABLE TO ALL WHO SINCERELY SEEK THE KINGDOM OF GOD FIRST IN CHRIST AS MATTH. 6:33 SAYS, "BUT SEEK FIRST THE KINGDOM OF GOD AND HIS RIGHTEOUSNESS, AND ALL THESE THINGS SHALL BE ADDED TO YOU."

AGAIN IN MY CASE, FOR ALMOST TWO YEARS, ALREDY BEING FILLED WITH THE HOLY SPIRIT OF WISDOM, POWER, LOVE AND UNDERSTANDING, STILL I DID NOT EXPERIENCE, NOR DID I KNOW ABOUT THIS!!!.

I MUST FRANKLY SAY THAT I CANNOT REALLY EXPLAIN THIS. IN MY LIFE I REMEMBER TO HAVE NOTICED JUST A FEW, MAYBE 2 OR 3 PERSONS THAT DURING THE WORSHIP SEEMED TO BE MAKING STRANGE GESTURES WITH THEIR LIPS AS I DO, AND REJOYCING FROM IT. THE ONLY THING I CAN SAY IS THAT JESUS IN JOHN 7:38 SAYS"HE WHO BELIEVES IM ME, AS THE SCIPTURES HAS SAID, OUT OF HIS HEART WILL FLOW RIVERS OF LIVING WATERS ". SO WHAT CAN I SAY THEN? BUT IF THE LORD WANTS TO BLESS US MORE WITH THE HOLY SPIRIT' S VARIOUS GIFTS AND BLESSINGS, WELL WE MAY AS WELL TAKE ANYTHING HE GIVE US!

SO TO YOU, WHO ARE READING THIS, BE ENCOURAGED AND EXPECTANT AS YOU STAND WITH A GRACIOUS AND WONDERFUL SAVIOUR, WE MUST CONTINUE TO ABIDE IN HIM IN REVERENT SUBMISSION [JOHN 15].

CONCLUDING PLEASE OBSERVE THAT THE SCRIPTURES GIVE US MANY REFERENCES ON THE LORD'S PROMISE TO PROVIDE US WITH THE HOLY SPIRIT AND ALSO WITH LIVING AND SATISFYING WATERS; WE ALSO SEE THE HOLY SPIRIT REFERRED TO AS BREATH AND WIND [ISA. 12:3; 44:3; 55:1; JOHN 4:10-14; 7:37-38. EZ. 37; JOHN 3:8; ACTS2: 1-4]. MOREOVER BREATHING IS CENTRAL FOR LIFE; I HAVE HEARD IN FACT THAT IN THE HEBREW LANGUAGE, LIVING MEANS BREATHING!

BUT LET US LOOK TOGETHER AT ISA. 12:2-3, " BEHOLD, GOD IS MY SALVATION, I WILL TRUST AND NOT BE AFRAID; 'FOR YAH, THE LORD IS MY STRENGTH AND SONG; HE ALSO HAS BECOME MY SALVATION.' "THEREFORE WITH JOY YOU WILL DRAW WATER FROM THE WELL OF SALVATION."

AND FINALLY JOHN 7:37-38, " ON THE LAST DAY, THE GREAT DAY OF THE FEAST, JESUS STOOD AND CRIED OUT, SAYING, "IF ANYONE THIRSTS, LET HIM COME TO ME AND DRINK."HE WHO BELIEVES IN ME, AS THE SCRIPTURE HAS SAID, OUT OF HIS HEARTS WILL FLOW RIVERS OF LIVING WATER."

THE LORD CERTAINLY KNOWS WHAT HIS CHILDREN NEED
AND AT TIME DESERVE, BUT ALWAYS FROM HIS
GRACE AND FOR HIS GLORY, AMEN!!!

****

THIS SECOND STORY IS JUST A LITTLE ACCOUNT THAT
AGAIN HAPPENED TO ME ABOUT 16 YEARS AGO', DURING
MY BIBLE COLLEGE YEARS. NOW ITS CONTEXT IS AROUND
THE TIME I WAS INVOLVED IN MUCH EVANGELISM, IN
PARTICULAR IN MY ATTEMPT TO EVANGELIZE AN ENTIRE
IRANIAN FAMILY WITH GOD'S TRUTH OF SALVATION. I
THINK THAT MY EFFORTS WERE QUITE DEAR TO ME DUE
TO THE FACT ALSO THAT THE STATE OF IRAN HAS ALWAYS
BEEN IN MY HEART; FOR THIS REASON ALSO, I WAS
WITHOUT DOUBT TOO INVOLVED WITH THIS FAMILY. AS
ALREADY MENTIONED IN THIS BOOK, AN ITALIAN LADY
FRIEND HAD INTRODUCED TO ME THIS IRANIAN LADY,
WHOM I SHALL REFER TO HER AS MRS A..

AS YOU KNOW SINCERE MOTIVATION AND LOVE IS VITAL
IN OUR MINISTRY AS THE MOST FAMOUS VERSE IN THE
BIBLE SHOWS US: JOHN 3:16.

THIS IS CLEARLY EVIDENCED IN 2 JOHN 1, "TO THE ELECT
LADY AND HER CHILDREN, WHOM I LOVE IN TRUTH, AND
NOT ONLY I, BUT ALSO THOSE WHO HAVE KNOWN THE
TRUTH ".

MRS A. CAME FROM A NOBLE FAMILY IN IRAN, VERY
WELL KNOWN BOTH IN POLITICS AS WELL AS IN THE
RELIGIOUS CIRCLE. HER HUSBAND HAD BEEN A CLOSE
GENERAL OF THE KING, AND SHE HAD ALSO RELATIVES
WHO HAD BEEN MINISTERS, AND AT LEAST ONE AS
AN AYATOLLAH TO THE KING. NOW I HAD LEARNED THAT
SHE HAD LOST HER HUSBAND IN THE IRANIAN
REVOLUTION IN 1979, WHO WAS TO BE MORE PRECISE
EXECUTED AFTER BEING TORTURED. NOW IT FOLLOWED
THAT BECAUSE OF POSSIBLE PERSECUTION TO HER AND
HER FAMILY, SHE WENT TO LIVE IN SAUDY, WHERE HER
UNCLE WAS AN AMBASSADOR.

I AM ALSO AWARE THAT HER TWO CHILDREN ATTENTED
PRIVATE SCHOOLS HERE IN UK, AND I BELIEVE THAT NOW
THEY BOTH HAVE GOOD AND PROFESSIONAL JOBS IN
LONDON. I BELIEVE TO HAVE MET MRS A. IN 94; SHE WAS
VERY ATTRACTIVE AND ELEGANT; BUT ALSO SHE WAS
NOT HAPPY IN HER LIFE, NEITHER WAS SHE A CHRISTIAN.
SHE WAS NOT WORKING, AND SUFFERED FROM BACK
PAINS AND DEPRESSION. SADLY SHE WAS NOT LIVING A
GODLY MORAL LIFE TOO. WHEN I MET HER, HER
CHILDREN WERE STILL IN UNIVERSITY, SHE LIVED WITH
HER SON, AND HAD A TENANT/FLAT MATE. AS YOU
PROBABLY HAVE ALREADY GUESSED I DID LIKE HER TOO,
DESPITE I WAS VERY CAREFUL IN MY CONDUCT WITH
HER. I HAVE ALSO TO ADMIT THAT I WAS A LITTLE
ENCHANTED BY HER MIDDLE EASTERN BEAUTY, BEING
ALSO MUCH YOUNGER THAN NOW.

ANYHOW I HAD TAKEN UPON ME AS A BURDEN TO GIVE HER AN HAND AND TO WIN HER AND HER FAMILY FOR JESUS!

SO I OFTEN USED TO TAKE HER OUT FOR COFFES AND SOMETHING TO EAT; ALSO I OFTEN SPENT TIME IN HER PLACE FOR TEA AND FOR MEALS. I REMEMBER TAKING HER AT TIME TO THE WEST END, AND FEELING A LITTLE CONCERNED FOR OUR SAFETY AS SHE WOULD BE WEARING LONG AND THICK CHAINS AROUND HER NECK MADE OF PURE 14 AND 18 CARAT GOLD. I GUESS IT WAS JUST A DIFFERENT MENTALITY, AND SHE EXPLAINED TO ME ONCE THAT WHEN SHE WAS LIVING IN SAUDY ARABIA, IT WAS CUSTOM THERE TO CARRY GOLD FROM BANK TO BANK ON PEOPLE'S SHOULDERS. HAVING WARNED HER THAT LONDON WAS QUITE A DIFFERENT CONTEXT, SHE BEGAN TO HIDE HER NECKLACES/CHAINS UNDER HER CLOTHES.

NOW IN TRUE HONESTY, I MUST SAY THAT I WAS FREQUENTING THIS LADY TOO OFTEN, DESPITE I WAS ATTENDING CHURCH SERVICES EVEN 3 TIMES PER WEEK. ENDEED THINGS WERE NOT RIGHT; I WAS TOO CLOSE TO HER, AT LEAST EMOTIONALLY! MY MENTALITY WAS AND STILL IS THAT EVEN CADDLES BETWEEN A MAN AND A WOMAN NOT ENGAGED, ARE NOT ALLOWED; SOMEHOW, THESE WOULD BE ALREADY PHYSICAL AND SPIRITUAL IDOLATRY AND ADULTERY, IN TURN LEADING TO GREATER SEXUAL SINS AND BONDAGE! IN FACT I HAD SAT A FEW TIMES TOO CLOSE TO HER AND ONE DAY, I WAS REALLY DOWN, ALMOST ON THE BORDER TO

FEELING DEPRESSED, I KNEW THAT IT WAS THE LORD
WHO HAD CRUSHED MY SPIRIT IN CHASTENING ME TO
TEACH ME TO MANTAIN A CERTAIN DISTANCE WITH THIS
LADY, IN LINE WITH JAMES 1:27, " PURE AND UNDEFILED
RELIGION BEFORE GOD AND THE FATHER IS THIS: TO VISIT
ORPHANS AND WIDOWS IN THEIR TROUBLE, AND TO
KEEP ONESELF UNSPOTTED FROM THE WORLD." IN FACT
AS I WAS PRAYING ABOUT IT, ONE MORNING EARLY
WHEN I WAS STILL LYING IN BED, I FELT AS THE SPIRIT OF
GOD CAME OUT OF ME, AND BEGAN TO HOVER OVER
ME, AND THEN I FELT AS BEING SMACKED BY HIM! I HAVE
TO SAY THAT IT WAS RATHER SCARING, BUT AT LEAST
THAT REALLY HELPED ME TO UNDERSTAND WHY I HAD
BEEN SO DOWN TWO DAYS EARLIER. BUT THIS WAS NOT
ALL HOWEVER, I STILL WAS SOCIALISING WITH HER TOO
OFTEN.

THANK GOD, SOMETHING LATER IN THE FUTURE
HAPPENED TO ME THAT GAVE ME MORE STRENGTH AND
UNDERSTANDING, ENABLING ME TO GET CLOSER TO THE
LORD, AND TO LEAVE MUCH OF THE TASK TO SAVE HER
TO THE HOLY SPIRIT. YES IT HAPPENED THAT ONE
EVENING I WAS ABOUT TO CALL HER AND TO GO TO VISIT
HER. I WAS JUST ABOUT TEN MINUTES WALK FROM HER
HOUSE. HAVING ENTERED INTO A TELEPHONE BOX TO
CALL HER, SUDDENLY I WAS TRYING TO UNDERSTAND
WHY WAS I GOING TO SEE HER SO OFTEN, WHAT WAS
REALLY THE DESIRE OF MY HEART?

NOW AS I WAS ASKING MYSELF THIS QUESTION, IN MY MIND I BEGAN TO ANSWER MYSELF IN THIS WAY << I AM GOING THERE TO....>>; BUT SUDDENLY THE VOICE OF THE LORD, WHO WAS REALLY GUIDING ME IN THIS, COVERED AND TOOK OVER MY THOUGHTS WITH HIS OWN LIVING WORDS AND VOICE IN THIS WAY << ...TO WORSHIP HER.....>>.

AS YOU KNOW, AND TO MY SHAME THEN, THIS WAS PURE IDOLATRY! A BREECH TO THE FIRST COMMANDMENT " AND GOD SPOKE ALL THESE WORDS SAYING: 'I AM THE LORD YOUR GOD, WHO BROUGHT YOU OUT OF THE LAND OF EGYPT, OUT OF THE HOUSE OF BONDAGE.'YOU SHALL HAVE NO OTHER GODS BEFORE ME " [EX. 20:1-3].

IN HIS MERCY THE LORD HAD BEEN VERY GRACIOUS TO ME AT THAT PARTICULAR TIME. NOW AS I THINK BACK AT THIS EXPERIENCE AND I TRY TO RECALL THE NATURE OF THE LORD'S VOICE, I WOULD LIKE TO MAKE AND SHARE THIS PARTICULAR REFLECTION WITH YOU. FIRSTLY I MUST CONFESS THAT I FELT ALMOST LIKE AN IDIOT, IN COMPARISON TO HIS WISDOM! HIS VOICE AND WORDS WERE JUST PURE DIVINE WISDOM, MUCH BEYOND ANY HUMAN CAPABILITY! SECONDLY THE NATURE OF HIS VOICE AND WORDS WERE ALSO PURE AND DIVINE LOVE/MERCY TOWARDS ME, AGAIN FAR BEYOND ANY

HUMAN CAPABILITY! WELL, I AM SURE THAT YOU CAN IMMAGINE HOW THAT EVENING I CHANGED DIRECTION, AND INSTEAD OF CALLING HER I WENT TO CHURCH!

NOW I DO NOT REMEMBER EXCATLY WHETHER BEFORE THIS HAPPENED OR A LITTLE LATER, I REALLY AM NOT SURE NOW, THE LORD HAD SPOKEN TO ME AT ANOTHER TIME, AND IN THIS SAME CONTEXT. IT WAS, I BELIEVE ON A SATURDAY MORNING THAT I HAD JUST GONE FOR A RUN, AND I WAS COMING BACK HOME ON A BUS, WITH SOME BAGS OF SHOPPING WITH ME. NOW I WAS STILL A LITTLE TOO BOTHERED ABOUT THIS FRIENDSHIP, AND EVEN ANY POSSIBLE CONNECTION WITH MY MISSIONARY DESIRE TOWARDS THE COUNTRY OF IRAN. SO THERE I WAS SITTING ON BUS N.16 TRAVELLING IN KILBURN, NORTH LONDON. IN MY MIND WERE GOING THROUGH THOUGHTS ABOUT MRS A., AND THE WAY IN WHICH I WOULD BE TRAVELLING TO IRAN IN THE FUTURE TO DO GOD'S WORK. PLEASE BE REALISTIC, BUT IN MY YOUNGER MIND, MY REASONING WAS THAT SHE WAS CONNECTED WITH MANY IMPORTANT PEOPLE IN HER COUNTRY, AND IF CONVERTED, AFTER HER FRIENDS AND RELATIVES IN IRAN WOULD HAVE POSSIBLY FOLLOWED HER EXAMPLE. WELL..... I AM SURE THAT YOU CAN AGREE WITH ME THAT IT DID SOUND GREAT!

BUT HOWEVER MAN'S TOUGHTS ARE NOT GOD'S TOUGHTS AND HIS WAYS ARE MUCH HIGHER THAN OURS AND THESE WERE NOT PART OF HIS PLAN. IN FACT

THANKS BE TO GOD, ISA. 55: 8-9 TELLS US THAT, " 'FOR MY THOUGHTS ARE NOT YOUR THOUGHTS, NOR ARE YOUR WAYS MY WAYS,' SAYS THE LORD.'FOR AS THE HEAVENS ARE HIGHER THAN THE EARTH, SO ARE MY WAYS HIGHER THAT YOUR WAYS, AND MY THOUGHTS THAN YOUR THOUGHTS."

SO IN THIS STATE OF MIND THINKING EVEN ABOUT A POSSIBLE MARRIAGE WITH HER [AS SHE INDEED MAY HAVE WANTED TO MARRY ME ALSO], SUDDENLY I DECIDED THAT THIS WAS NOT THE RIGHT WAY TO GO ABOUT IT, AND NEITHER SHE WAS GOING TO BE MY WIFE, NO MATTER HER POSITION IN THE IRANIAN SOCIETY; BUT IN THE CASE GOD'S WORK IN HER COUNTRY WAS GOING TO BE DONE THROUGH THE CHURCH CONTEXT, EVEN COSMOPOLITAN AS OUR CHURCH IS, AND BY THE SPIRIT OF THE LORD AS HE WOULD LEAD! AS YOU KNOW WHEN WE LOVE AND CARE FOR OTHER PEOPLE WE NEED TO BE VERY CAREFUL IF WE WANT TO AVOID SERIOUS COSEQUENCES FOR US AND OTHERS, SINCE LOVE IS A VERY DEEP EMOTION.

AS I HAD MADE UP MY MIND ON THIS THAT SUDDENLY THE VOICE OF THE LORD CAME TO ME IN MY BOSOM IN ENGLISH, AS I ALSO WAS THINKING IN ENGLISH. THIS TIME IT WAS THE FATHER SPEAKING, AND THIS IS WHAT HE TOLD ME IN HIS CLEAR AUDIABLE LIVING VOICE << EH,

EH, YOU ARE GOING TO DO GREAT THINGS MY SON >>. WE ALL KNOW THAT SOMETIMES GOD ALLOW US TO GO THROUGH ALL KIND OF EXPERIENCES IN ORDER TO MATURE OUR CHARACTERS IN VARIOUS TESTS OF LIFE. JUST LOOK AT THE LIVES OF JOSEPH AND MOSES, AS BOTH WERE VERY RICH WITH GOOD AND DIFFICULT LIFE SITUATIONS [GEN. -EXODUS]. BY THE WAY, AT THE MOMENT IT HAS BEEN LONG TIME SINCE I HAVE SEEN THIS LADY'S CHILDREN, AS I ASLO DO NOT THINK THEY WERE INTERESTED TO KEEP IN TOUCH WITH ME, AND AS FOR THEIR MOTHER, I WAS TOLD THAT SHE HAD COMMITTED SUICIDE WITH AN OVERDOSE OF HER REGULAR SLEEPING OR ANTI DEPRESSION TABLETS, AND I HAVE NOT SEEN HER SINCE THAT REPORT, THAT IS FOR PERHAPS ALMOST 10 YEARS NOW.

NO MATTER WHO WE ARE AND WHAT WE DO, THE WORD OF THE LORD STILL GOES ON HOWEVER. NOW WHAT I STILL, IF I MAY DARE TO SAY SO, REMEMBER AND PRAISE ABOUT THE VOICE OF GOD THE FATHER, WAS [BELIEVE IT OR NOT], HIS SENSE OF HUMOR, HIS TOTAL WISDOM, TOTAL SOVEREIGNTY OF HISTORY INCLUDING OURS, AND THE FATHERLY CHARACTER/NATURE OF HIS VOICE, WHICH ALSO HAD REMINDED ME OF [IN A MUCH SMALLER HUMAN SCALE], OF MY HUMAN FATHER, WHO FAR FROM BEING PERFECT, WAS A CARING, LOVING AND STRICT FATHER; BY THE WAY HE PASSED AWAY IN 2000, AND ON THIS COMING FEBR. 2012, HE WOULD HAVE COMPLETED

101 YEARS IN FEBR. 2012, THAT IS IN A FEW WEEKS TIME AS I WRITE.

WELL TO GOD BE THE GLORY FOR HIS WONDERFUL FELLOWSHIP WITH US, THE ONLY IMMANUEL GOD WITH US, AS FROM THE SCRIPTURES I HAD UNDERSTOOD THAT IT WAS THE LORD JESUS WHO HAD BEEN PLEASED TO REVEAL TO ME HIS FATHER, AND FOR BOTH OF THEM TO MAKE THEIR HOME IN ME [MATTH 11:25-27; JOHN 14:23], AS THEY DO IN ALL BELIEVERS WHO OBEY GOD'S COMMANDMENTS!!!

SO LET US END THIS PASSAGE WITH JOHN 14:23, "JESUS ANSWERED AND SAID TO HIM, 'IF ANYONE LOVES ME, HE WILL KEEP MY WORD; AND MY FATHER WILL LOVE HIM, AND WE WILL COME TO HIM AND MAKE OUR HOME IN HIM."

****

I BELIEVE THAT WHAT FOLLOWS IS AN EXTRAORDINARY SHORT NARRATIVE THAT AGAIN, IF IT HAD NOT BEEN JUSTIFIED BY THE SCRIPTURES, I WOULD HAVE BEEN VERY RELUCTANT TO WRITE ABOUT IT. NOT ONLY THIS BUT I WOULD LIKE TO ADD THAT IT IT IS MY HOPE THAT THIS LITTLE STORY WILL HELP SHEDDING MUCH LIGHT ON A VERSE OF THE SCRIPTURES WHICH IS GIVEN AMOST ALWAYS OTHER INTERPRETATIONS OTHER THAN WHAT I

AM ABOUT TO TELL YOU HERE, WHICH ALSO REFLECTS MORE THE LITERAL SENSE OF THE TEXT. THIS VERSE IS FOUND IN EPH. 6:16, THAT IS"ABOVE ALL, TAKING THE SHIELD OF FAITH WITH WHICH YOU WILL BE ABLE TO QUENCH ALL THE FIERY DARTS OF THE WICKED ONE. "

BY THE WAY MOST OF US KNOW THAT IN PAST HISTORY FIERY DARTS WERE OFTEN USED IN BATTLES; WELL DO BE AWARE THAT THE DEVIL STILL USES THEM, BUT THESE ARE INVIVIBLE TO THE VISIBLE EYES, AND SO I THINK EVEN MOST CHRISTIANS DO NOT UNDERSTAND IT!

THIS SHORT ACCOUNT OF EVENTS THAT I AM ABOUT TO WRITE TO YOU IS SET HERE IN LONDON, AND TAKE US BACK, I THINK TO 1996 WHEN I WAS FINISHING MY EVENING CERTIFICATE IN OUR CHURCH BIBLE COLLEGE. AS I HAVE ALREADY MENTIONED IN THIS BOOK, BY NOW THE LORD HAD ALREADY BEGAN TO TAKE ME THROUGH VARIOUS EXPERIENCES IN THE SPIRIT, BOTH WITH HIM AND WITH EVIL SPIRITS TO EQUIP ME AND BUILD ME UP IN MY MISSIONARY CALLING. NOW I HAD STARTED THIS BIBLE CLASS IN 95 BY ATTENDING ONE EVENING PER WEEK, AND IN 96 I WAS ABLE TO ATTEND TWO EVENINGS PER WEEK. AT THE SAME TIME I WAS SUPPORTING MY MINISTRY AND STUDY BY WORKING IN A RESTAURANT IN CENTRAL LONDON NEAR PICCADILLY. AS MENTIONED BEFORE IN THAT TIME I WAS VERY ZELOUS IN PRAYER, INTERCESSION, SINGING AND EVANGELISM, AS WELL AS HELPING OTHER PEOPLE IN OTHER PRACTICAL WAYS.

NOW ONE DAY IT HAPPENED THAT I WAS WORKING IN THE RESTAURANT, BUT I DO NOT REMEMBER EXCATLY IF WE WERE IN THE LUNCH SHIFT OR IN THE DINNER ONE; BUT THAT DOES NOT REALLY MATTER. NOW I RECALL THAT I WAS GOING THROUGH A PARTICULAR PROBLEM, OR BASICALLY THERE WAS A SMALL ISSUE THAT I HAD TO RESOLVE WITH THE MANAGER. FOR MY BENEFIT THIS MANAGER WAS RATHER A GENTLEMAN, ENGLISH, INTELLIGENT, BROUGHT UP IN A CHRISTIAN CONTEXT, AND MAY THE LORD BLESS HIM, HE WAS THE ONE TO HELP ME AND ENCOURAGE ME TO GO TO BIBLE COLLEGE FULL TIME BY ALLOWING ME TO WORK ONLY IN THE EVENING IN THE NEXT YEARS; ALSO HIS ASSISTANT, AN IRANIAN YOUNG LADY, WHOM I HAD KNOWN FOR A FEW YEARS, WAS QUITE HELPFUL TOO. BASICALLY THEY WERE PEOPLE THAT I COULD TALK TO WITH A CERTAIN CONFIDENCE. SO IT HAPPENED THAT I WAS WAITING FOR THE RIGHT MOMENT TO TALK TO THE MANAGER TO TRY AND RESOLVE THIS SMALL ISSUE THAT WAS BOTHERING ME.

TO MY MEMORIES I THINK MOST PEOPLE AND MANY THEOLOGIANS SEE THESE "FIERY DARTS" AS DEMONIC TEMPTATIONS, LIES, EVIL AND NEGATIVE THOUGHTS THROWN AT OUR MINDS. BUT PLEASE DO NOT GET ME WRONG; THE DEVIL DOES THAT TOO! WE COULD SAY THAT NOW AS IN THE GARDEN OF EDEN, IT IS ABOUT HEEDING GOD'S WORD, OR OURS AND THE DEVIL!

I CANNOT AVOID HERE SHOWING THAT SPIRITUAL
WEAPONS ARE VERY POWERFUL, AS IN WHAT THE
PROPHET ISAIAH SAYS IN 11:4, ON THE SECOND COMING
OF THE MESSIAH, SOMETHING THAT OUR WORLD NEEDS
SO BADLY, AND THAT ALL CHRISTIANS ARE LOOKING
FORWARD TO, " BUT WITH RIGHTEOUSNESDS HE SHALL
JUDGE THE POOR, AND DECIDE WITH EQUITY FOR THE
MEEK OF THE EARTH; HE SHALL STRIKE THE EARTH WITH
THE ROD OF HIS MOUTH, AND WITH THE BREATH OF HIS
LIPS HE SHALL SLAY THE WICKED."

JUST TO ADD TO THIS, JUST A FEW WEEKS AGO' IN MY
CHURCH, SOMEBODY PROPHESIED POINTING TOWARDS
MY DIRECTIONS. WHAT I CAN TELL YOU IS THAT I
RECIEVED IT FOR MYSELF ANYHOW; AND DO KNOW THAT
AS HE SPOKE THE SHATTERING WORD OF GOD, I FELT AS
LIKE A SHIELD OF STONE AND UNBELIEF 'CAME OUT OF
ME', IT SHIFTED AWAY. HIS ENCOURAGEMENT WAS
ABOUT PRAYING AND INTERCEDING WITH THE
ASSURANCE THAT THINGS WILL CHANGE/SHIFT [I THINK
IN MY LIFE]!

BUT SEE WHAT JEREMIAH SAYS IN 23:29, "'IS NOT MY
WORD LIKE A FIRE?' SAYS THE LORD, ' AND LIKE A
HAMMER THAT BREAKS THE ROCK IN PIECES? "

NOW BACK TO MY STORY, THE MANAGER CAME
UPSTAIRS, AND WHEN I SAW HIM CLOSE TO ME, I

PREPARED MYSELF TO SPEAK TO HIM. SUDDENLY AS I WAS DOING SO, SOMETHING VERY UNUSUAL OCCURRED THERE THAT TRIED TO STOP ME TO COMMUNICATE WITH HIM. WHAT HAPPENED WAS THAT, AS I WAS ABOUT TO APPROACH HIM, ON MY RIGHT HAND SIDE I SAW SOMETHING EXTRAORDINARY! PLEASE TRY TO PICTURE NOW THIS FOLLOWING BRIEF DESCRIPTION OF MINE JUST HERE BELOW:

AT ABOUT TWO METERS AWAY FROM ME, AND IN THE AIR AT ABOUT TWO METERS HIGH, I SAW SOMETHING THAT LOOKED LIKE BRIGHT, YELLOWISH ROUND SPOTS. THESE APPEARED AS STANDING IN THE AIR LIKE FORMING THE STRUCTURE OF A CIRCLE; THIS CIRCLE WAS ABOUT FIFTEEN CM. IN DIAMETER, AND EACH SPOT WOULD DISTANCE ITSELF FROM EACH OTHER PERHAPS 1-3 CM, BEING PROBABLY IN ALL ABOUT TEN-TWELVE SPOTS FORMING THIS CIRCLE " OF FIRE "!

STRAIGHT AWAY THIS RECALLED TO MY MIND THE PASSAGE OF EPH 6:16 IN WHICH THE APOSTLE PAUL SAYS"ABOVE ALL, TAKING THE SHIELD OF FAITH WITH WHICH YOU WILL BE ABLE TO QUENCH ALL THE FIERY DARTS OF THE WICKED ONE ".

IN FACT, THANK GOD I HAD JUST STUDIED THE ARMOUR OF GOD AS PART OF THE MODULE "KNOW YOUR ENEMY ", DURING THE EVENING CERTIFICATE AT OUR BIBLE COLLEGE.

NOW, SUDDENLY THE SPOTS HAD DISAPPEARED AND I FELT AS THEY WERE THROWN AT ME INSIDE AND WITHIN MY CHEST/BOSOM.

IN THAT VERY MOMENT I WAS CHANGED, I FELT MY COURAGE AND STRENGTH, AND CONFIDENCE WERE GONE, AND I WAS GRABBED WITH FEAR; I WAS NO MORE IN CONDITION TO SPEAK TO MY MANAGER!

DURING THE FIRST FEW SECONDS EVEN MY HEART WAS GOING AGAINST ME, PERHAPS UNDER THE DIRECTION OF THE EVIL AND LYING ONE, AND SO IN MY THOUGHTS I WAS TRYING TO JUSTIFY/EXPLAIN TO MYSELF THAT I WAS FEELING IN THIS WAY BECAUSE MY WORKING POSITION WAS ONLY THAT AS A WAITER, AND THE ENGLISH LANGUAGE WAS NOT MY FIRST LANGUAGE....; AND SO IN THIS WAY I WAS, IN IGNORANCE, ONLY DESPISING MYSELF AND INCREASING THE DAMAGING WORK OR THE DEVIL IN ME, WHO WANTED TO STOP ME FROM SPEAKING AND SUCCEDING IN GOD'S WORK. BUT THESE NEGATIVE THOUGHTS LASTED ONLY FEW SECONDS IF NOT LESS!

AND QUITE RIGHTLY SO, AS I UNDERSTAND NOW MORE THAN THEN IN 1996, WHAT I REALLY DID WAS "CASTING DOWN ARGUMENTS AND EVERY HIGH THING THAT EXALTS ITSELF AGAINST THE KNOWLEDGE OF GOD, BRINGING EVERY THOUGHT INTO CAPTIVITY TO THE

OBEDIENCE OF CHRIST," AS PAUL TEACHES US IN 2 COR. 10:5. IN FACT, SUDDENLY AS I RECOGNISED THE FIERY ARROWS OF THE WICKED ONE, AND HIS ATTACK AGAINST ME, I PROCEEDED BY THE WORD OF THE LORD, AND BY TAKING THE SHIELD OF FAITH, THAT IS THE NAME OF JESUS, WITH ALL MY FAITH AND POWER I CURSED THE DEVIL IN MY HEART AND THOUGHT [NOT IN AUDIABLE WORDS, AS I WAS IN THE MIDDLE OF THE RESTAURANT, AS I HAD TO BE WELL BEHAVED,].

TO BE MORE PRECISE I ALSO USED THE SWORD OF THE SPIRIT AS IN V. 17," AND TAKE THE HELMET OF SALVATION, AND THE SWORD OF THE SPIRIT, WHICH IS THE WORD OF GOD;"

STRAIGHT AWAY I FELT FREE, SOMETHING OPPRESIVE, THAT IS THE FIERY DARTS OF THE ENEMY HAD COME OUT OF ME! MY COURAGE AND STRENGTH HAD COME BACK TO ME!!!

AFTER ONLY A FEW MINUTES, I WAS ABLE TO CONVERSE WITH MY MANAGER AND SUCCESSFULLY RESOLVE MY ISSUE, THANKS BE TO GOD!

THOUGH I FOUND ONLY ONE THEOLOGIAN DURING A SMALL RESEARCH OF MINE, WHO SUPPORTS THIS LITERAL

SENSE OF THIS VERSE, THE BIBLE OFTEN SPEAK OF FIRE, SUCH AS IN: PS.7:13; ISA.66:15;MATTHEW 5:22; JUDE 7; 1 COR.1: 3,15; 2 PETER 3:7.

LET US NOW FIRSTLY OBSERVE THIS IMPORTANT WARNING FROM THE LORD IN MATTH. 5:22, "BUT I SAY TO YOU THAT WHOEVER IS ANGRY WITH HIS BROTHER WITHOUT A CAUSE SHALL BE IN DANGER OF THE JUDGMENT. AND WHOEVER SAYS TO HIS BROTHER, 'RACA!' SHALL BE IN DANGER OF THE COUNCIL. BUT WHOEVER SAYS, 'YOU FOOL!' SHALL BE IN DANGER OF HELL FIRE." AND NOW THIS, IN A WAY, GREAT ENCOURAGEMENT IN ISAIAH 66:15-16, " FOR BEHOLD, THE LORD WILL COME WITH FIRE AND WITH HIS CHARIOTS, LIKE A WHIRLWIND, TO RENDER HIS ANGER WITH FURY, AND HIS REBUKE WITH FLAMES OF FIRE. FOR BY FIRE AND BY HIS SWORD THE LORD WILL JUDGE ALL FLESH; AND THE SLAIN OF THE LORD SHALL BE MANY."

IMPORTANT PASSAGES ARE ALSO REV. 9; AND VERSE 17:16.

*** BUT PLEASE VERY IMPORTANTLY, SEE THE DEVIL BURNING JOB'S POSSESSIONS WITH FIRE IN JOB 1:11-16, THOUGH, UNAWARE, THE PEOPLE THERE THOUGHT IT TO BE 'THE FIRE OF GOD', "...AND THE LORD SAID TO SATAN, 'BEHOLD ALL THAT HE HAS IS IN YOUR POWER; ONLY DO NOT LAY A HAND ON HIS PERSON.' SO SATAN WENT OUT FROM THE PRESENCE OF THE LORD....AND A MESSENGER

CAME TO JOB AND SAID...WHILE HE WAS STILL SPEAKING, ANOTHER ALSO CAME AND SAID, 'THE FIRE FROM GOD FELL FROM HEAVEN AND BURNED UP THE SHEEP AND THE SERVANTS, AND CONSUMED THEM, AND I ALONE HAVE ESCAPED TO TELL YOU!"

SCARY, IS NOT IT, IF IT HAD NOT BEEN FOR OUR IMMANUEL? ***

***VERY INTERESTING INDEED, AND IT DOES MORE JUSTICE TO THE TEXT IN EPHESIANS 6:16!!!

WELL FOR SURE WE KNOW THAT THE DEVIL HAS NOT RETIRED JUST JET, AND SO SITTING BACK AND COLLECTING HIS PENSION, BUT IT MAYBE THAT HE IS ALSO INVOLVED IN SOME CONTEMPORARY FIRES ROAMING ON EARTH LIKE SOME RECENT ONES IN AUSTRALIA AND USA!!!

THUS AGAIN WE MUST BE VERY CAUTIOUS BEFORE WE AGREE WITH MANY OTHER INTERPRATATIONS.

NOW, HAVING TOLD YOU THIS REVEALING EXPERIENCE, WHICH I HOPE YOU WILL TREAUSURE AND MAKE USE OF IT BENEFICIALLY, I JUST WANT TO MAKE A FEW COMMENTS TO HELP YOU FOR OUR COMMON ANALYSES.

FIRSTLY THE WEEK BEFORE THIS EXPERIENCE I WAS LEAD BY THE LORD IN GIVING A SPECIAL OFFERING OF ABOUT 20% OF MY WEEKLY WAGES, AND ALTHOUGH, I CANNOT REMEMBER EXCATLY, I DO RECALL TO HAVE ASKED HIM TO LET ME SEE THE INVISIBLE, AS TO INCREASE MY UNDERSTANDING IN RELATION TO MY CHRISTIAN LIFE AND THE WORLD.

NOTE THAT IN THE SCRIPTURES THE ELEMENT OF SACRIFICE IS CENTRAL, NOTHING IS FOR FREE! SALVATION COSTED THE LORD THE CROSS; AND ALL THESE GRACES THAT WE EXPERIENCE, IS BECAUSE OF THE CROSS TOO. WE ARE ALSO CALLED TO GIVE, AND SACRIFICE FOR HIM IN ORDER TO SHARE IN HIS BLESSINGS AND GLORY [2 COR. 9:1-12].

ANOTHER, IF NOT THE MOST IMPORTANT OBSERVATION I WOULD LIKE TO MAKE IS THAT, THIS SPIRITUAL ACCOUNT OF THE FLAMING ARROWS OF THE EVIL ONE WHICH I HAVE JUST DESCRIBED TO YOU, IT ACTUALLY DOES JUSTICE TO THE LITERAL TEXTUAL MEANING OF THE VERSE IN EPH. 6:16!!!

UNFORTUNATELY WHEN SOME THEOLOGIANS AND PASTORS DO NOT EXPERIENCE THESE, THEN THEY TEND TO GIVE THIS VERSE MORE METAPHORICAL MEANINGS, SUCH AS FOR EXAMPLE THAT THIS VERSE TELL US ABOUT DIFFERENT LIES THROWN AT US BY THE

DEVIL, AND WHICH WE CAN ESTINGUISH WITH THE SHIELD OF FAITH WICH IS THE WORD OF GOD.

HOWEVER THIS ONLY WORKS FOR THE DEVIL WHO DOES NOT WANT US TO KNOW BOTH THE WORD OF GOD, AND WHAT HE KNOWS THAT WE DO NOT KNOW ABOUT HIM!

* FOR YOUR INTEREST PLEASE BE INFORMED OF THIS:

1-IN THE WEEK THAT I WAS TAKING SOME NOTES ON THIS TOPIC FROM A BOOK THAT AGREED WITH THIS INTERPRETATION OF MINE, I SUFFERED A MUCH HIGHER LEVEL OF STRESS THAN USUAL.

2-AS I HAD JUST FINISHED TO TAKE THESE MUCH MORE ACCURATE NOTES FROM THIS BOOK IN A OLD LIBRARY, THOUGH I WAS NOT AWARE, THE LORD MUST HAVE BEEN ON MY LEFT HAND SIDE, AS I HEARD HIS VOICE SAYING TO ME " BRAVO ". BUT I THINK BECAUSE I DID NOT HUMBLE MYSELF, NOR WAS I GREATFUL ENOUGH TO HIM, FOR THE FIRST TIME IN THIS APPLICATION, THESE NOTES GOT STUCK IN THE OUTBOX OF MY SMART PHONE AND THEN DISAPPEARED! I HAD TO WRITE THEM AGAIN THE NEXT DAY!

3-THE NEXT DAY I WAS CROSSING A LARGE HIGHWAY TO GO TO THIS LIBRARY, WHICH HAD THREE LINES OF CARS MOVING ONE WAY, AND OTHER THREE LINES OF CARS GOING THE OPPOSITE WAY. JUST BEFORE CROSSING, I FELT DISTRACTED TO LOOK ON THE WRONG SIDE OF THE ROAD, AND THEN JUST IN TIME I REALISED THAT THREE LINES OF CARS WERE POINTING TOWARDS ME FROM THE OTHER SIDE; I FELT AS IF THE DEVIL HIMSELF THROUGH A SERIOUS OF CIRCUMSTANCES ORCHESTRATED BY HIM, LIKE IN A SIEGE AGAINST ME, HAD JUST CAUSED ME TO TURN MY FACE TO THE WRONG DIRECTION, TRYING TO GET ME RUN OVER! *

NOW NO DOUBT THAT HE IS ALSO A LIER AND IN FACT WE HAVE OTHER VERSES THAT TELL US SO. HOWEVER WITH RESPECT TO OTHERS' INTERPRETATIONS, THE WORDS IN THIS VERSE SEEM TO BE QUITE PARTICULAR AND YOU MAY WANT TO KEEP IN MIND ALSO WHAT I HAVE JUST WRITTEN HERE, AS IT REFLECTS THE WRITTEN TEXT WELL!

ANOTHER REFLECTION THAT I WOULD LIKE TO PRESENT TO YOU IS THE FACT THAT WHEN WE DO NOT KNOW THE SCHEMES OF THE DEVIL, AND NEITHER HIS WEAPONS, NOT ONLY IS MORE DIFFICULT FOR US TO DEFEND OURSELVES, BUT EVEN WORSE, WE CAN FURTHER DAMAGE OURSELVES. WHAT I MEAN IS THAT WE CAN

BECOME PARTNER WITH THE DEVIL IN FURTHER HURTING OURSELVES, ACCORDING TO HIS EVIL SCHEMES.

FOR EXAMPLE IF I HAD NOT FREED MYSELF IN THE WAY WHICH I DID, THAT IS WELL AND WITHOUT BAD CONSEQUENCES TO ME, I PROBABLY WOULD HAVE HAD TO LOOK FOR SOMEKIND OF DRUGS TO CURE MY FEELINGS OF OPPRESSION AND FUTURE DEPRESSIONS AND FRUSTRATIONS, WHEN REALLY THESE WOULD HAVE NOT BEEN THE APPROPRIATE BEST CURE. AND SO IN THIS WAY BRINGING INTO MYSELF FINANCIAL LOSSES AS WELL AS SIDE EFFECTS FROM DRUGS, WITHOUT REALLY SOLVING THE PROBLEM AT ITS ROOTS TOO! THUS NOT BEING ABLE TO FULFILL GOD'S PERFECT WILL FOR MY LIFE AS WITH NO DOUBT HAPPENS TO MANY MEN OF GOD, INCLUDING MY UNCLE, WHO HAD BEEN A PATIENT OF A PSCHIATRIC HOSPITAL FOR OVER FORTY YEARS AND THE LAST FEW YEARS IN HIS LIFE IN A PROTECTED FAMILY HOUSE.

PLEASE ALSO OBSERVE THIS LAST REFLECTION OF MINE.

AT MY YOUNG AGE, WHEN I WAS PERHAPS FIFTEEN YEARS OLD, I BEGAN AT TIMES TO SUFFER CERTAIN FEELINGS OF OPPRESSION, SUCH AS I HAVE DESCRIBED IN THIS ACCOUNT WHEN THE EVIL ONE THREW HIS FIERY DARTS AT ME. UNFORTUNATELY, BECAUSE OF MY IGNORANCE OF THE SCRIPTURES, [SEE ALSO THE RELATED ISSUES OF THE LOCAL CHURCHES, ETC, AS MENTIONED IN THE INTRODUCTION], BECAUSE I COULD NOT DEFEND MYSELF, AS I DO NOW, I ADDED TO THE DAMAGING

WORK OF THE DEVIL WITH FRUSTRATIONS, DEPRESSIONS, ISOLATION, ETC... AND AS YOU HAVE READ IN THE INTRODUCTION, AT THE AGE OF SEVENTEEN I WAS A PATIENT OF AN INSTITUTION FOR "SPIRITUAL DEPRESSION", THANK GOD ONLY FOR TWELVE DAYS. THEN AFTER A YEAR I ALSO GOT RID OF THE "SPIRITUAL DRUGS " I WAS GIVEN. ALTHOUGH DRUGS FREE, I SUFFERED OF DEPRESSION FOR YEARS TILL PERHAPS THE EARLY NINETIES; AT TIMES A DEEP DEPRESSION WHICH AT THE AGE OF TWENTYFIVE, AS I HAVE ALREADY TOLD YOU, LEAD ME TO TAKE AN ALMOST SUICIDIAL JOURNEY TO INDIA EITHER TO FIND THE WILL OF LIVING OR DEATH, AS I ALMOST HAD NO MONEY EVEN FOR THIS FIVE WEEK JOURNEY; AFTERWARDS I STARTED MY LIFE AGAIN, BACK HERE IN LONDON ONLY WITH THREE DOLLARS!

PEHAPS IN MY LITTLE WAYS, EVEN MYSELF I HAVE PAYED A PRICE IN ORDER TO REVEAL TO YOU THIS DEMONIC WEAPONS DESCRIBED IN EPH. 6:16. BUT NOW I OFTEN REJOICE IN THE LORD MY SAVIOUR!

MOSTLY HOWEVER I AM IMMENSELY GREATFUL TO OUR LORD JESUS CHRIST THAT DURING THESE YEARS PROTECTED ME FROM THE SCHEMES OF THE EVIL ONE TO DESTROY ME AND CAUSE ME EVEN TO TRY TO LET MYSELF DYE OF HUNGER IN INDIA. NOT ONLY THIS I ALSO GIVE HIM ALL THE GLORY FOR HIS HOLY SPIRIT AND FOR HAVING REVEALD TO ME THESE DEMONIC WEAPONS,

AND THE POWER/AUTHORITY TO DEFEAT THEM; IN FACT FOR MANY YEARS THE DEVIL DOES NOT ATTACK ME ANYMORE AS HE KNOWS IT WILL NOT BE CONVENIENT TO HIM, AS I WILL SERIOUSLY REBUKE AND CURSE HIM TO HIS LOSS AND SHAME!!!

FOR OUR LORD IS NOT ONLY CREATOR AND SAVIOUR BUT ALSO HEALER, AND WE ARE TO USE THE POWER OF THE SHIELD OF FAITH THAT IS THE NAME OF JESUS, AND SPEAK IT OUT.

SO GLORY BE TO GOD WHO ALSO HELP US TO RESIST THE DEVIL FROM ALL OF HIS OTHERS SCHEMES AGAINST US, SUCH AS HIS LIES, TEMPTATIONS AND ACCUSATIONS TO BRING US DOWN [EPH. 6:11; REV. 12:10]. ALSO THANK BE TO OUR GOD, FOR HIS BLOOD WHICH NEVER LOOSES ITS POWER AS EVIDENCED IN REV.12:11, "AND THEY OVERCAME HIM BY THE BLOOD OF THE LAMB AND BY THE WORD OF THEIR TESTIMONY, AND THEY DID NOT LOVE THEIR LIFE TO DEATH." AMEN.

****

I AM CONCLUDING THIS CHAPTER AND INDEED ALL THIS LITTLE AUTHOBIOGRAPHY OF MINE, WITH ONE OF THE MOST, IF NOT INDEED THE MOST BEAUTIFUL EXPERIENCE IN MY LIFE TILL TODAY EXCEPT THE ONE FROM HAVING RECIEVED HIS SALVATION, IF I MAY SAY

SO. NOW THIS IS A SHORT ACCOUNT THAT OCCURED HERE IN LONDON I THINK A FEW YEARS AFTER I FINISHED BIBLE COLLEGE, PERHAPS IN 2001-2003, BUT I REMEMBER CLEARLY THAT IT WAS IN THE MONTH OF NOVEMBER OR DECEMBER, AS IN THAT TIME I HAD TAKEN TO A CONFERENCE IN WEMBLEY ARENA A FRIEND THAT I WAS TRYING TO HELP.

I WANT TO BIGIN TO REFLECT ON JESUS SHINING DURING THE TRANSFIGURATION, I WOULD LIKE TO BIGIN WITH BY SAYING THAT NOT ONLY IS THIS SO, BUT JESUS ALSO BROUGHT BRIGHTNESS, LIGHT, AND SPLENDOUR INTO THE OLD TESTAMENT; HE SHONE THROUGH IT AS WELL AS IN OUR LIVES IN OUR TIMES!

NOW AT THAT TIME I WAS STUDYING BY CORRISPONDENCE FOR MY BA [HON.] IN THEOLOGY WITH THE OPEN THEOLOGICAL COLLEGE FROM CHELTENHAM IN UK; AND IN THE EVENING I WOULD BE WORKING IN A RESTAURANT IN PICCADILLY, AS WELL AS BEING INVOLVED IN CO-PASTORING A SMALL SATELLITE CHURCH OF KT, OUR MAIN CHURCH, UNDER THE LEADERSHIP OF THE MAIN SATELLITE PASTOR AND HIS WIFE.

I ALSO USED TO CONTINUE ATTENDING OUR MAIN CHURCH, AS THE GREATER PART OF MY EVANGELISTIC/APOSTOLIC WORK HAD AND STILL HAS

A MORE INTERNATIONAL FOCUS AND SCOPE,
WHILE MOST PEOPLE IN THE SATELLITE BRANCH WERE OF
SIERRA LEONE NATIONALTY.

I THINK, AT LEAST FOR MY OWN CAPACITY, MY WEEK
WAS RATHER BUSY; QUITE RIGHT SINCE HE IS A GOD OF
GLORY AND LIKES US TO SHARE IN IT AND BE ACTIVE
BRINGING MORE GLORY TO HIM.

AS FOR MANY OF US, THERE WERE PRESSURES AT WORK,
IN THE CHURCH, IN THE STUDY, AND IN THE FAMILY.
ALSO, TO GOD BE THE GLORY, I WAS QUITE BUSY IN
REACHING OUT PEOPLE; FEELING THEREFORE BOTH THE
BURDEN OF GOD'S CALLING IN MY LIFE, AS WELL AS THE
GREAT JOY, FUN AND SATISFACTION IN WITNESSING TO
OTHERS, HELPING THEM TO BE ROOTED IN OUR MAIN
CHURCH OR IN ONE OF OUR SATELLITES, AND MOSTLY IN
CHRIST. RIGHT NOW I CANNOT REMEMBER THE PERSON
WHO WROTE THAT MISSIONARIES DO NOT NEED A
HOME, THEY ONLY NEED A REFUGE; IN FACT BY THE
GRACE OF GOD HERE IN LONDON, FROM 1995 I HAVE
ONLY SPENT TWO EVENINGS IN MY HOME, BECAUSE I
HAD SOME FEVER AND A BAD COLD, OTHERWISE I HAVE
BEEN EITHER WORKING OR OUTSIDE AVAILABLE FOR
OTHER PEOPLE! AND WE HAD BETTER BE BUSY DOING HIS
WORK SINCE OUR SAVIOUR IS BOTH LOVING AND READY
TO JUDGE!

I REMEMBER IN THIS PERIOD I WAS ALSO WITNESSING TO A YOUNG, OFTEN HOMELESS GIRL. SOMETIMES SHE WOULD LOOK DIRTY AND BE SMELLY TOO. A FEW TIMES I WAS ABLE TO TAKE HER TO CHURCH ALSO, AND ONCE AS I HAVE ALREDY SAID, TO A CONFERENCE. FROM HER I KNEW THAT HER FATHER HAD ABBANDONED HER WHEN SHE WAS ONLY FOUR YEARS OLD, AND HAVING PROBLEMS WITH HER MOTHER, SHE HAD LEFT HER HOME IN SCANDINAVIA AS A YOUNG TEENAGER. CLEARLY WHAT I CAN SEE NOW EVEN BETTER THAN BEFORE IS HER FAMILY'S NEED FOR UNITY THROUGH THE DEDICATION OF HER PARENTS TO EACH OTHER AND TO GOD, A LACK THAT SADLY WE SEE EVERYWHERE AND AT ALL LEVEL OF SOCIETY!

AND SO IN VARIOUS WAYS I WAS TRYING TO HELP HER, ESPECIALLY TO CONVINCE HER TO JOIN A WOMAN FELLOWSHIP; IN ADDITION, AT LEAST ONCE I WAS ABLE TO SPEAK ON THE PHONE TO HER MOTHER, WHO HAD TOLD ME THAT HER DAUGHTER DID NOT WANT TO COME BACK HOME. AT THE SAME TIME I WAS BEGINNING TO FEEL THE PRESSURES A LITTLE TOO MUCH; OFTEN AT WORK, WE WERE SHORT OF STAFF, AND PERHAPS AT TIMES WE HAD TO WORK IN HARD CONDITIONS. ANYHOW IN ALL THIS STATE OF THINGS, AT TIMES I BEGAN TO FEEL WEAK AND FEELING LIKE FAINTING, AS IF MY HEAD WAS FAILING ME, AND SO REACHING ALMOST THE POINT TO FALL ON THE FLOOR. I BELIEVE, AS ALSO

MY DOCTOR HAD TOLD ME AFTER SOME TESTS, IT WAS JUST BECAUSE OF PROBABLY TOO MUCH STRESS.

SOMETIMES AGO' A BROTHER OF MINE, WHO IS A DOCTOR TOLD ME THAT IT IS HEALTHY TO BE IN THE LIGHT, SUCH AS THE SUNSHINE, OR EVEN BY THE WATERS, SINCE THESE REFLECT LIGHT; SOMETHING THAT I FIND VERY INTERESTING AS NOT ONLY THE LORD JESUS SAYS THAT IS THE LIGHT OF THIS WORLD, BUT ALSO WE CAN FIND VARIOUS LINKS TO THIS IN THE O.T.

BUT LET US LOOK AT NUM. 5:24-25 AND APPROPRIATE IT FOR US AND OUR LOVED ONES," 'THE LORD BLESS YOU AND KEEP YOU; THE LORD MAKES HIS FACE SHINE UPON YOU, AND BE GRACIOUS TO YOU; THE LORD LIFT UP HIS COUNTENANCE UPON YOU, AND GIVE YOU PEACE'." AMEN! YES THE ABOVE IS NEEDED AGAINST ALL STRESS, SICKNESS, AND UNJUSTICE IN THIS WORLD.

AND SO DURING ONE EVENING SOMETHING VERY UNUSUAL AND BEAUTIFUL HAPPENED TO ME!!!

IT MUST HAVE BEEN ON A SUNDAY NIGHT AFTER CHURCH, THOUGH I AM NOT PERFECTLY SURE. AS USUALLY AFTER THE SERVICE, I WOULD BE GOING TOWARDS CENTRAL LONDON TO FIND OPPORTUNITY TO TALK WITH PEOPLE, AND ESPECIALLY MUSLIMS. IN THAT PERIOD I WOULD OFTEN BE SEEING A MAN FROM YEMEN WHO OFTEN WAS LONELY BEING SICK WITH A BLOOD CONDITION, AND ALSO THIS SCANDINAVIAN GIRL, AS

WELL AS OTHER PEOPLE. THAT NIGHT, HOWEVER I HAD
COME ACROSS AN INTERESTING MAN FROM SINGAPORE;
HE WAS CARRYING A ROCKSACK AND WAS HOMELESS. I
BEGAN TO WITNESS TO HIM THOUGH HIS SPOKEN
ENGLISH WAS NOT GOOD; I MARVELLED AT HIM AS
I COULD SEE THAT HE HAD A SPECIAL GOOD NATURE AND
COUNTENANCE. AS I THINK OF HIM, I WONDER WHAT
HAD HAPPENED TO HIM IN THE PAST, AS WELL AS
WHAT WILL HAPPEN TO HIM IN THE FUTURE. IS HE
GOING TO BECOME A PASTOR? WELL TIME WILL TELL.
CERTAINLY LIFE HAS NEVER BEEN AND IS NOT EASY FOR
ANYONE IN HUMAN HISTORY!!!

I CANNOT AVOID SAYING THAT MOSES, THOUGH LIVED IN
THE OLD TESTAMENT, IS EVEN TODAY FOR US LIVING IN
THE NEW TESTAMENT TIMES OF GRACE AND OF THE
HOLY SPIRIT, A GREAT INSPIRATION AND CHALLENGE;
JUST LOOK AT THE FOLLOWING CONTENT IN NUM. 12:6-
8, " THEN HE SAID, 'HEAR NOW MY WORDS: IF THERE IS A
PROPHET AMONG YOU, I, THE LORD, MAKE MYSELF
KNOWN TO HIM IN A VISION; I SPEAK TO HIM IN A
DREAM. NOT SO WITH MY SERVANT MOSES; HE IS
FAITHFUL IN ALL MY HOUSE. I SPEAK TO HIM FACE TO
FACE, EVEN PLAINLY, AND NOT IN DARK SAYINGS; AND HE
SEES THE FORM OF THE LORD. WHY THEN WERE YOU
NOT AFRAID TO SPEAK AGAINST MY SERVANT MOSES? ' "

IT IS WONDERFUL, IS NOT IT?

ANYHOW I HAD DECIDED TO TAKE HIM TO MACDONALD FOR A MEAL, WHERE ALSO THIS SCANDINAVIAN GIRL WAS. AND SO WITH THE GRACE OF GOD, I WAS ABLE TO SHARE A MEAL WITH THEM BOTH. IT WAS DIFFICULT TO SEE THIS SCANDINAVIAN GIRL EATING, AS I KNEW THAT SHE WOULD CHEW THE FOOD AND THEN PUT IT IN A PIECE OF PAPER AND REJECT IT. A DOCTOR FRIEND OF MINE TOLD ME THAT IT WAS BECAUSE SHE WAS SUFFERING FROM A PSYCOLOGICAL CONDITION THAT WAS AFFECTING HER SOCIAL BEHAVIOUR. WELL I DID SPENT SOME GOOD MOMENTS WITH THEM; THE MAN FROM SINGAPORE WAS GREATFUL TO ME AS HE HAD A NOBLE HEART, BUT AFTER THAT EVENING, I CONFESS THAT I NEVER SAW HIM AGAIN, BUT I AM SURE THAT YOU CAN NOW JOIN ME IN PRAYER WITH ME AS YOU READ THIS, THAT, IF HE HAS NOT JET, SOON, HE SHALL KNOW THE LORD AND BE USED BY HIM IN HIS GLORIOUS MINISTRY WITH GOOD KNOWLEDGE AND UNDERSTANDING, AMEN [2 COR. 3].

ON THE CONTRARY AT TIMES I STILL SEE THIS YOUNG LADY, THOUGH I TALK TO HER MUCH LESS AS I HAD UNDERSTOOD THAT SHE DID NOT WANT TO CHANGE HER LIFE JET, NEEDING THEREFORE MORE TIME, PRAYER AND ESPECIALLY "GUIDANCE " BY THE HOLY SPIRIT HIMSELF! IN THIS WAY WE CAN AVOID WASTING TOO MUCH TIME FOCUSING ON THE WRONG PEOPLE TOO; BUT EVEN TODAY [7-11-11], AS I PRAY AND YOU READ WHEN YOU WILL, PLEASE JOIN ME IN A PRAYER OF YES AND AMEN, THAT SOON THIS YOUNG LADY SHALL COME TO KNOW

GOD AS HER REAL FATHER, AND ALSO BE MENTOR BY GOOD AND OLDER CHRISTIAN WOMEN, AMEN.

SO IN THE SAME WAY I WOULD LIKE TO COMMENT THAT SOMEHOW WITH THESE SAME IMPLICATIONS AND FATHERLY CONCERN WE ARE INSTRUCTING NON-BELIEVING CHRISTIANS AS WE TRY TO EVANGELISE THEM.

ANYHOW I AM SURE YOU HAVE A LOT TO TELL ME OFF AS YOU READ THIS BOOK OF MINE, BUT I DO NOT THINK THAT, DESPITE ALL MY WEAKNESSES, YOU COULD SAY THAT I AM NOT GLOBALLY MINDED! AND QUITE RIGHTLY WE NEED TO BE SO!

THEN AS USUALLY I MUST HAVE LEFT THE PLACE OF OUR MEETING LATE THAT EVENING, PERHAPS AFTER HAVING WITNESSED TO OTHER PEOPLE TOO. NOW THAT EVENING I MUST HAVE ARRIVED HOME LATE MAYBE AROUND MIDNIGHT OR LATER. IT HAPPENED THAT WHEN I CAME INTO MY ROOM THAT, AS AT TIMES WE CAN ALL HAVE SOME DEEP NEEDS OR GO THROUGH A TIME OF PARTICULAR DISTRESS, I ALSO FELT UNDER A PARTICULAR PRESSURE TO CALL ON THE LORD. SUDDENLY, AT THE SAME TIME AS I WAS ALMOST FAINTING ON THE FLOOR BECAUSE OF WEEKNESS, AND SO I WAS SOMEHOW BOWING WITH MY BODY, THAT I SAW THE SPIRIT OF THE LORD ENTERING INTO MY ROOM THROUGH THE WALL ON MY LEFT AT A SUPERNATURAL SPEED! YES THE HOLY SPIRIT!

AND WE KNOW THAT INDEED JESUS, WHO IS ALSO THE PREACHER PER EXELLENCE, HE GOES WHEREVER HE WISHES, SO THAT MORE GLORY IS BROUGHT TO THE FATHER!

NOW AS HE ENTERED, HE MANIFESTED HIMSELF IN MY ROOM, AND FOR THE FIRST TIME IN MY LIFE HE ALLOWED ME TO SEE HIM FACE TO FACE, AND I AM GLAD THAT I WAS LOW AND BOWING IN MY PHYSICAL PERSON AND NOT STANDING UP, WHILE LOOKING AT THE FACE OF THE ANCIENT OF DAYS, DIRECTLY AND NOT TO A PROFILE OF HIS FACE AS I HAD SEEN HIM BEFORE. HE ONLY APPEARED TO ME PERHAPS JUST FOR 2-3 SECONDS. HIS APPEARANCE WAS JUST AS A DRAWING OF HIS FACE, THOUGH WITH VERY FEW INSIDE DETAILS. OBVIOUSLY WHEN YOU SEE HIM, YOU ALSO RECOGNISE HIM! YOU WILL REMEMBER IN FACT JOHN 10:4-5, IN WHICH THE LORD JESUS TELLS US THAT WE KNOW AND FOLLOW HIS VOICE AS THAT OF OUR SHEPERD: "AND WHEN HE BRINGS OUT HIS OWN SHEEP, HE GOES BEFORE THEM; AND THE SHEEP FOLLOW HIM, FOR THEY KNOW HIS VOICE. JET BY NO MEANS WILL FOLLOW A STRANGER, BUT WILL FLEE FROM HIM, FOR THEY DO NOT KNOW THE VOICE OF STRANGERS.' "

NOW NONE OF US SPOKE, WE ONLY LOOKED AT EACH OTHER, I IN AWE, AND HE IN HIS FAITHFUL MERCY. AS I

BEHELD HIM IN REVERENCE, I KNEW HE WAS THE SAME ONE AS HAD APPEARED TO THE PATRIARCH IN THE OLD TESTAMENT, AS WELL AS OUR RESURRECTED SAVIOUR, WHO APPEARED IN THE NEW TESTAMENT, AND ALSO SOMETIMES EVEN TODAY TO PEOPLE, AND SO I JUST IDENTIFIED MYSELF IN " THIS " AND REALLY " HIS " HISTORY.

JUST A FEW COMMENTS, NOW FROM THE MEMORY OF HIS FACE I STILL CAN SEE THAT HE BOTH REFLECTED DIVINITY AS WELL AS ROYALTY; HE ALSO LOOKED YOUNG AND NOT OLD, IF I MAY SAY SO IN THE LIMITATION OF OUR HUMAN LANGUAGE; HE REFLECTED LOVE, JUSTICE AND TRUTH; HE WAS WORTHY OF DEMANDING ALL REVERENCE; HIS FACE REFLECTED COMPLETE SHALOM: PEACE, PROSPERITY, FREEDOM, SAFETY, SECURITY, PERFECTION, COMPLETENESS,WISDOM AND UNDERSTANDING; IN HIM THERE WAS NO LUCK OF CONSECRATION, CONFIDENCE AND UNITY, NEITHER WAS THERE ANY SIGNS OF DESPAIR AND FRAGMENTATION; HE REFLECTED ALL THAT PEOPLE AND SOCIETY COULD EVER NEED AND LONG FOR!!! [HEBR. 1:12; GEN 1; REV. 22].

AS I REFLECT MORE ON THIS, I THINK THAT LIKE THE HOLY SPIRIT, WE NEED TO INTERFERE MORE WITH PEOPLE AND LOVE (NOT LUSTING) THEM IN FREEDOM.

MOREOVER ONE OF THE THINGS THAT STROKE ME MOST IN THIS EXPERIENCE WAS THE FACT THAT HIS FACE

APPEARED TO ME AS COMPLETELY AND PERFECTLY
ROUND IN HIS CIRCUMPHERENCE, WHICH ALSO
REMINDED ME OF THE ROUND SHAPE OF THE PLANETS.
NO DOUBT EVEN PLANETS ARE MEANS OF THE GRACE OF
GOD, AND SO ALSO SIGNS AND SIGNALS POINTING TO
BOTH GOD AND MEN [CF GEN. 15:5]. PERHAPS THIS
COULD ALSO BE A SIGN OF HIS UNIVERSAL INTENTION
AND DIMENSION OF SALVATION AND SOVEREIGNTY IN
THE UNIVERSE [CF. MATTH. 17:2; REV. 1:16].

AT THIS POINT LET US BE BLESSSED BY SEEING TOGETHER
REV. 1:16-17, "HE HAD IN HIS RIGHT HAND SEVEN STARS,
OUT HIS MOUTH WENT A SHARP TWO-EDGED SWORD,
AND HIS COUNTENANCE WAS LIKE THE SUN SHINING IN
ITS STRENGTH. AND WHEN I SAW HIM, I FELL AT HIS FEET
AS DEAD. BUT HE LAID HIS RIGHT HAND ON ME, SAYING
TO ME, ' DO NOT BE AFRAID; I AM THE FIRST AND THE
LAST."

IN THIS WAY WHEN MANY OF US BEGIN TO LOOK AT THE
EXPRESSION OF " SHALOM " IN THE FACE OF THE
SAVIOUR, TO HIS GLORY WE HAVE STARTED A PROCESS
OF REGENERATION, RESTORATION, AND REALLY WE HAVE
ALREADY BECOME A NEW CREATION [2 CHRON. 7:14; PS.
24:6; HEB.12:2; 2COR. 5:17].

IN ADDITION I WOULD LIKE TO TELL YOU THAT TO ME HE
LOOKED AS A SOVEREIGN AND AN AWESOME WARRIOUR,
THE CURVED, OR MORE LIKE, THE "SWOLLENESS" OF THE

SHAPES OF HIS CHEEKBONES WERE ROUNDISH AND VERY
PROMINENT ON HIS FACE. HIS APPEARENCE INSPIRED
AND DEMANDED FEAR, REVERENCE AS WELL AS
REFLECTED INFINITE FATHERLY AND DIVINE LOVE AND
GRACE!!!

BASICALLY WE WOULD HAVE NOT LIKED TO DISAGREE
WITH HIM!!!

WELL I DO NOT WANT TO BE IRONIC, BUT I WANT TO
ALLOW MYSELF TO USE A BIT OF SENSE OF HUMOR, AND
DARE TO SAY, OR ASK IF HE AND US REALLY LOOK
EVANGELICAL? I DO NOT REALLY KNOW WHAT TO SAY TO
THAT MYSELF!?!

FURTHER IT IS AT THIS POINT AND ON THE LOVE OF GOD
THAT I WOULD LIKE TO MAKE ANOTHER LITTLE
COMMENT. ABOUT FIFTEEN YEARS AGO' I WAS A
STUDENT PASTOR IN ANOTHER SATELLITE CHURCH OF
OUR MAIN CHURCH. NOW DURING THE SERVICE, OR JUST
BEFORE THE WORSHIP, I HAD GONE OUT TO EVANGELISE
IN THE SURROUNDING AREA SOMETIMES BY MYSELF,
AND AT OTHER TIMES WITH OTHERS. THIS TIME WITH
GOD'S GRACE I HAD BROUGHT BACK A HOMELESS MAN
TO THE CHURCH. HE STAYED WITH US IN THE SERVICE,
AND HAD TEA AND COFFE AFTERWARDS; AND I NEVER
SAW HIM AGAIN AFTERWARDS. WELL THAT NIGHT AS I
WAS RESTING THE LORD IMPRESSED ON ME, PERHAPS

JUST FOR LESS THAN ONE HOUR OR SO, HIGHER LEVELS OF HIS DIVINE LOVE FOR THIS POOR MAN. A POURING OF HIS SUPERNATURAL AND DIVINE LOVE FILLED MY HEART AND MIND, SO MUCH THAT IT CAUSED ME TO WEEP LIKE A BABY FOR THIS HOMELESS MAN.

BUT JUST THINK FOR A MOMENT ABOUT THE LOVE OF GOD FOR PEOPLE, FOR THE CHURCH, HIS BRIDE, SO THAT HE GAVE HIS ONLY SON? AND WHAT ABOUT HIS JELOUSY AS CREATOR AND HUSBAND? I KNOW, WE JUST CANNOT HANDLE THIS, WE NEED HIS HELP!!!

JUST THINK HOW SATAN HATES THE JEALOUSY OF GOD, ALSO FROM THIS SMALL ACCOUNT OF MINE AS FOLLOWS. JUST A FEW WEEKS AGO' AN IMPORTANT PASTOR FROM BOGOTA CAME TO MINISTER TO OUR CHURCH AT THE SEVEN PM SERVICE. HE SPOKE FROM THE BOOK OF THE PROPHET NAHUM, ON THE JUDGMENT OF ASSYRIA WHO HAD CAPTURED THE NORTHERN KINGDOM OF ISRAEL, AND THE NEED FOR US TO OBEY THE LORD IF WE WANT TO AVOID GOD'S PUNISHMENT. WELL WHEN HE SPOKE ABOUT GOD'S JEALOUSY [1:2], BY MISTAKE HIS TRANSLATOR SAID 'ZELOUS' INSTEAD OF 'JEALOUS'! AT THE END OF THE SERVICE I WAS ABLE TO TALK TO THEM AND EXPLAIN THIS TO BOTH OF THEM. PLEASE NOTE THAT WHEN I ARRIVED TO MY HOME, THERE WAS SUCH A SCARING AND SINISTER/DEMONIC PRESENCE JUST IN FRONT OF MY HOUSE THAT THE ALL PLACE OUTSIDE LOOKED DIFFERENT, AND DESPITE MY MANY EXPERIENCES I WAS REALLY SCARED!

IN A LIKEWISE EXPERIENCE, ABOUT FEW YEARS AFTER, AFTER HAVING EVANGELISED TO THREE NON-CHRISTIAN WOMEN ON A BUS, THAT SAME NIGHT, WHILE RESTING AND STILL AWAKE, THE LORD HIT ME AGAING WITH TOUCHES OF HIS EXTRAORDINARY COMPASSIONATE AND OVERWHELMING DIVINE LOVE, SO THAT AGAIN I WAS LED TO WEEP FOR THEM, TO FEEL DEEP EMOTIONS FOR THEM, AS CUT OFF/SEPARATE AND IN NEED FOR THE LORD OUR SAVIOUR. DESPITE IN BOTH THESE OCCASIONS I WAS SUFFERING AS I WAS WEEPING AND HURTING, AS THE HOLY SPIRIT WAS CAUSING ME TO IDENTIFY IN A SUPERNATURAL MANNER WITH THE STATE OF THEIR MISERY AND RECKNESS, FOR THIS MAN AND THESE THREE LADIES, I, BEYOND ALL DOUBT COUNT THESE 'DIVINE/HUMAN IDENTIFICATION A TREMENDOUS PRIVILEDGE!

BASICALLY SINCE THE LORD HAS COME DOWN TO US, NOW, WITH THE HOLY SPIRIT TOO, WE HAVE TO COME DOWN ON THEM!

A NICE COMMENT IS NOT IT? EASIER FOR GOD/JESUS TO SEEK AND FIND US!

I KNOW THAT YOU KNOW THAT THESE FEELING WERE NOT REALLY FROM ME; IN FACT I THINK TO HAVE EXPERIENCED THIS HIGH LEVELS OF DIVINE LOVE AND EMOTIONS THIS TWO TIMES ONLY! AS HUMANS, AND ALSO LIVING HERE ON EARTH WITH ALL THAT IS

GOING ON, WE COULD NOT CONTAIN THESE
SUPERNATURAL FEELINGS, NEITHER COULD WE COPE
WITH THEM!

AS IN HEBR. 12, ALSO PAUL ENCOURAGES US TO PUSH
FORWARD TO SHARE ON THE GLORY OF GOD HERE IN
PHIL. 3:13-14, "...BUT ONE THING I DO, FORGETTING
THOSE THINGS WHICH ARE BEHIND AND REACHING
FORWARD TO THOSE THINGS WHICH ARE AHEAD, I PRESS
TOWARDS THE GOAL FOR THE PRIZE OF THE UPWARDS
CALL OF GOD IN CHRIST JESUS. "

AS I WRITE AT THIS MOMEMENT, LONDON HAS JUST
BEEN SHOCKED BY THREE DAYS OF RIOTS CAUSING
PHYSICAL INJURIES AS WELL AS BUILDING ON FIRE AND
DESTROYED. LIKE EVERY WHERE IN THE WORLD
LONDONERS AS WELL AS YOUNG PROPLE NEED BOTH
LOVE AND GRACE, BUT CERTAINLY ALSO AND ESPECIALLY,
THEY NEED FEAR/REVERENCE OF BOTH PARENTAL AND
STATE AUTHORITY, AND ULTIMATELY OF GOD HIMSELF,
SO THAT IT MAY GO WELL WITH US ALL. MY REFLECTION
IS THAT BOTH SOCIETY AND THE CHURCH IN IT, IN ORDER
TO FEAR GOD, NEED TO KNOW AND REVERE HIS WORD
FIRST!

BUT SEE 2 PETER 1:20-21, WHICH ON THE CONTRARY
TELLS THAT "KNOWING THIS FIRST, THAT NO PROPHECY
OF SCRIPTURE IS OF ANY PRIVATE INTERPRETATION, FOR
PROPHECY NEVER CAME BY THE WILL OF MAN, BUT HOLY

MEN OF GOD SPOKE AS THEY WERE MOVED BY THE HOLY
SPIRIT."

WELL CERTAINLY THIS MAIN EXPERIENCE IN SEEING THIS
SPECIAL APPEARENCE OF THE LORD, BROUGHT GREAT
JOY AND MANY OTHER BLESSINGS IN MY LIFE, AND ALSO
CONTINUOUS COURAGE TO SERVE HIM IN MY MINISTRY.
AT THE SAME TIME I HOPE THAT IT HAS BLESSED YOU
TOO. INDEED IT IS MY FERVENT DESIRE AND PRAYER THAT
THIS ALL SMALL BOOK OF MINE WILL BE FOR YOUR
BENEFIT AND EDIFICATION, IN ALL POSSIBLE WAYS AS
YOU READ IT WITH THE HELP OF THE HOLY SPIRIT, AND
MEASURING STICK OF THE HOLY SCRIPTURES; IN FACT ALL
BOOKS, AS WELL AS OUR LIVES, MUST BE JUDGED BY THE
BIBLE, AS THE SUPREME DIVINE SOURCE OF AUTHORITY
[2 PETER 1:20-21]!

PLEASE DO FORGIVE ME OR EXCUSE ME IF I AM
AVOIDING WRITING A SEPARATE CHAPTER AS A
CONCLUSION FOR THIS BOOK. IN FACT I BELIEVE AND
RECOGNISE THAT THIS IS NOT MAINLY A BOOK ABOUT
ME, BUT MOST OF ALL, OF WHATEVER AMOUNT OF THE
CONTENT OF THIS BOOK CAN BE SEEN AND SAID, IT IS
MAINLY A BOOK ABOUT JESUS STILL LIVING AND
ACTING TODAY IN MY LIFE AS WELL AS IN THE LIVES OF
MILLIONS OF US! AND IN RECOGNITION OF ALL OUR
IMPERFECTIONS AND EVIL INTENTIONS AT TIMES, AND
WEAKNESSES, THOUGH IN HIS MERCY AND GRACE HE

PARTNERS WITH US AND SO SHARE OF HIS HONOUR
WITH US, HE ALONE IS THE CENTRE OF EVERYTHING!

IT IS BY HIS LOVE AND GRACE THAT HE HAS GIVEN US HIS
TRUTH IN THE BIBLE!

AS THE LORD JESUS WAS THE CENTRE OF BOTH THE OLD
TESTAMENT AND THE NEW, SO IT IS AND SHOULD BE
EVEN MUCH MORE ALSO TODAY, THE CENTRE OF
IMPORTANCE AND ATTENTION IN THE WORLD.

IN THIS WAY, WITH BENT KNEES AND HANDS UP TO GIVE
HIM ALL GLORY, I ADMIT, IN LINE WITH THE APOSTLE
JOHN, THAT REALLY THERE IS NEVER AN END AND A
CONCLUSION ABOUT THE BOOK ON THE LIFE OF THE
ACTIONS OF JESUS CHRIST; AND AS ALREADY SAID, ONLY
HE IS THE PREACHER PER EXELLENCE!

AND SO IN HUMBLE ADORATION AND FEAR OF GOD, I AM
LEAVING THIS BOOK OPEN WITH THE WORDS OF THE
BIBLE, BY THE BELOVED APOSTLE JOHN " AND THERE ARE
ALSO MANY OTHER THINGS THAT JESUS DID, WHICH IF
THEY WERE WRITTEN ONE BY ONE, I SUPPOSE EVEN THE
WHOLE WORLD ITSELF COULD NOT CONTAIN THE BOOKS
THAT WOULD BE WRITTEN. AMEN " [JOHN 21: 25]. AND
ALSO WITH THE WORDS OT THE BROTHER OF THE LORD "
NOW TO HIM WHO IS ABLE TO KEEP YOU FROM
STUMBLING, AND TO PRESENT YOU FAULTLESS BEFORE

THE PRESENCE OF HIS GLORY WITH EXCEEDING JOY, TO GOD OUR SAVIOUR, WHO ALONE IS WISE, BE GLORY AND MAJESTY, DOMINION AND POWER, BOTH NOW AND FOREVER. AMEN. "

[JUDE 24-25].

==================================

www.ingramcontent.com/pod-product-compliance
Lightning Source LLC
Chambersburg PA
CBHW072043280526
45788CB00006B/2160